SMART MEDICINE

FAMILY HEALTH JOURNAL

OTHER BOOKS IN THE SMART MEDICINE SERIES

Smart Medicine for a Healthier Child

Smart Medicine for Healthier Living

SMART MEDICINE

FAMILY HEALTH JOURNAL

JANET ZAND, N.D., L.Ac.

ROBERT ROUNTREE, M.D.

RACHEL WALTON, MSN, CRNP

ALLAN N. SPREEN, M.D., CNC

JAMES B. LAVALLE, R.Ph., N.D.

Avery
a member of
Penguin Group (USA) Inc.
New York

Most Avery books are available at special quantity discounts for bulk purchase for sales promotions, premiums, fund-raising, and educational needs. Special books or book excerpts also can be created to fit specific needs. For details, write Penguin Group (USA) Inc. Special Markets, 375 Hudson Street, New York, NY 10014.

AVERY

a member of
Penguin Group (USA) Inc.
375 Hudson Street
New York, NY 10014
www.penguin.com

Copyright © 2004 by Janet Zand
Portions of this book are taken from *Smart Medicine for Healthier Living*
by Janet Zand, Allan N. Spreen, and James B. LaValle and
Smart Medicine for a Healthier Child by Janet Zand, Rachel Walton,
and Robert Rountree.

ISBN: 1-58333-186-7

Printed in the United States of America
10 9 8 7 6 5 4 3 2 1

Book design by Mauna Eichner

CONTENTS

Introduction: How to Use This Book   vii

PART ONE

SMART MEDICINE BASICS
1

Introduction: The Nuts and Bolts
   of Smart Medicine   3
The Smart Medicine Cabinet   10
A Guide to Common Symptoms   14

PART TWO

CHILDREN'S GROWTH AND DEVELOPMENT RECORDS
19

Your Child at Birth   21
Children's Height and Weight Charts   26
Developmental Milestones   31
Diet Diary   32
Immunization Record   42
Well-Baby Visits   45

PART THREE
FAMILY HEALTH RECORDS
67

APPENDIX I
IMPORTANT DOCUMENTS
193

APPENDIX II
IMPORTANT NAMES AND NUMBERS
205

INTRODUCTION: HOW TO USE THIS BOOK

This is a journal that will help you to keep track of *all* the important information you need about your family's health and health care. There are places for recording information about children's growth and development, as well as the health care of all family members. The forms for recording this information are set up in a way that we hope will encourage you to combine the best of conventional medicine, herbal medicine, homeopathy, diet, nutritional supplementation, and other approaches for all the members of your family. Obviously, you may not have something to record in each category for each page, but this book is designed to give you the maximum flexibility in recording the things you need to know. Finally, there is space to attach important original documents, and an easy register for you to keep important names and numbers ready at hand.

When recording health information—whether about symptoms, responses to different treatments or other measures, or anything else—be as observant and specific as possible. For example, if you are experiencing pain, describe its nature in as much detail as you can. Is it sharp or dull? Does it stay at the same level or does it come and go? Exactly where are you feeling it? Make a note of things that seem to make symptoms better and things that seem to make them worse—heat, cold, activity, inactivity, consuming food or liquid, the time of day, or anything else you notice. Similarly, when you use any form of treatment, record observations of your responses as precisely as possible. This is particularly useful if you are using homeopathic remedies, the correct selection of which depends on what can seem like minute details of your symptoms and other factors. Record any questions you want to ask your health-care practitioner when they occur to you. Then, by bringing this book with you to your doctor appointments, you will have a detailed record that can help to ensure that nothing is overlooked and questions are not forgotten amid the bustle (and stress) of a health-care visit. This will help both you and your doctor in achieving the best results for you.

We recommend that you fill out the section for emergency numbers and any professionals you already see right away. Then, when you consult any new practitioners, add them to the list also. That way, should an emergency or illness arise, you will know exactly where to look for this information, and it will all be in one place.

PART ONE

SMART MEDICINE BASICS

INTRODUCTION: THE NUTS AND BOLTS OF SMART MEDICINE

The Smart Medicine philosophy is that the best approach to health and health care is an integrated one that considers *all* treatment possibilities and draws on what works. In our view, it is just as significant that a particular therapy has been used effectively for hundreds or thousands of years as it is that a scientific paper substantiates a particular approach. We believe that so-called natural healing therapies and conventional medical treatment can—and should—work together. In fact, more and more health-care professionals of all types are incorporating this understanding into their practices, and there are more multidisciplinary clinics in which medical doctors, naturopathic physicians, acupuncturists, nutritionists, homeopaths, chiropractors, and counselors work together in an integrated manner, treating the patient as a whole person.

Using a complementary approach to health care, we can draw on modern conventional medicine, natural medicine, and ancient healing traditions to find what is most effective and supportive in curing and preventing illness. This book is meant to be a unique resource that will enable you to record *all* of the information about your and your family's health histories in one place. As such, it will help you to implement an integrated approach to health care and to keep track of relevant observations about which types of treatments have worked for you.

The following are brief summaries of some of the modalities you may wish to call upon for health and healing.

CONVENTIONAL MEDICINE

When most Americans think of health care, they think of conventional medicine. It is without question the dominant approach to medicine in the United States today, and it permeates our basic understanding of sickness and health—often without our being aware of it. For example, many people think of health as being the absence of disease, and when they don't feel well, they are apt to ask, "Is there something I can take for this?" Both of these ideas reflect the assumptions of modern conventional medicine, which tends to be oriented toward identifying diseases and prescribing cures, usually in the form of drugs or, sometimes, surgical procedures. This is probably because most of us grew up with conventional medicine, also called "orthodox,"

"Western," or "modern" medicine. In the United States, conventional health care usually means a visit to your physician. Depending on the reason for the visit, your doctor may run tests, prescribe a drug, recommend dietary changes and exercise, refer you to a specialist or surgeon, or merely tell you to make sure to get extra rest and to drink lots of fluids.

Conventional medical science emphasizes the importance of the scientific method—logical study that produces reliable results that can be duplicated. In the last few decades, medicine has made progress that would have been unthinkable just three or four generations ago. The use of insulin injections has allowed people with diabetes to live long and relatively healthy lives; the discovery of antibiotics has improved the treatment and prognosis for people with bacterial and tubercular infections; the polio vaccine was developed and has largely eliminated this dreaded disease; and organ transplantation has become an accepted, viable treatment for certain conditions. Increasingly sophisticated diagnostic tools and advances in treatment have been developed. In addition, the course of conventional medicine has included the creation of huge drug companies, health-insurance programs, and government agencies like the National Institutes of Health. All of these developments have played a role in shaping the health-care system we know today.

Because of the many successes in the treatment of infectious diseases, the emphasis in medical research has now shifted toward the chronic and degenerative diseases, which remain less curable. Heart disease, the various forms of cancer, and acquired immune deficiency syndrome (AIDS) are among the health problems that pose the greatest challenges to medical science today. Since chronic and degenerative diseases are usually the cumulative result of many factors, rather than a reaction to a single agent, practicing preventive medicine—eating a healthful diet, exercising regularly, reducing stress, and making healthy lifestyle choices such as not smoking and limiting alcohol intake—is becoming more and more central to taking care of our health.

Many sophisticated diagnostic tools are available to medical doctors today. Some have long been familiar, such as the stethoscope, otoscope, and x-ray. More recent advances also include computerized axial tomography (CAT) scanners, magnetic resonance imaging (MRI), and other laboratory tests. Yet like all healing systems, conventional medical science evolved from a long tradition of careful observation. Even with the tremendous advances of the last century, the most important tool a conventional physician has is still his or her willingness to listen closely and observe carefully.

Physicians are here to help you make appropriate decisions, to work with you. Even if you favor a natural approach to health care, there may come a time when only conventional medicine has the cure you need. A physician who truly knows you and your medical history is a wonderful resource, especially in times of crisis. Unfortunately, with the advent of managed care and our increasing mobility, it is not always possible to consult a doctor with whom you have an ongoing relationship. That is one of the reasons for this book; it will enable you to keep records of treatment you have received in the past that you can take with you if you must see an unfamiliar doctor, so that he or she can get a clearer and more detailed picture of your health history.

There may be a time when your doctor recommends a comprehensive health-care program for you or another family member. A good doctor will work with you in formulating a regimen that is both effective and manageable. Make sure you fully understand all phases of any program your doctor is suggesting. Ask as many questions as

TIPS FOR CHOOSING A HEALTH-CARE PROVIDER

Whatever type of health professionals you consult, there are a few rules of thumb for ensuring a positive experience. Keep in mind the following:

• Choose a practitioner who keeps up to date with the latest treatments. New treatments are being developed all the time. This is especially true with new pharmaceutical drugs, which by definition do not have long histories of safe use. The side effects of drugs should be understood and carefully considered.

• Find a practitioner who is open-minded about natural and complementary therapies. A conventional medical doctor does not necessarily have to prescribe natural medicine (and an alternative practitioner may not be able to prescribe conventional drugs), but he or she should at least be willing to listen to your ideas and explore options. A practitioner who will work with you in taking an integrated approach to health care is invaluable.

• Find a practitioner who will work with you as a partner—who believes in making decisions *with* you, rather than *for* you.

• Choose a practitioner who is a good communicator—who not only can explain situations and treatments to you in a way you can understand, but who also really listens and responds to your questions and concerns.

• Choose a practitioner who looks at the big picture. It is essential to work with someone who does not look at you only as a case of a given illness or condition, but as a whole person.

• Find a practitioner who is willing to see you and interact with you as the intelligent, caring person that you are.

• While you want a doctor who is as well qualified and capable as possible, you also want someone who knows his or her limitations, and who is willing to call upon those with more expertise in a specific area if warranted.

• If a time ever comes when a practitioner no longer has your trust, it's probably time to make a change.

necessary. Don't just passively agree to diet, to take medication, or to make lifestyle changes that will be immensely difficult or perhaps even impossible to carry out. Airing your fears and concerns is an important part of your responsibility. Without your input, your doctor has no way of knowing that you find a program difficult or impossible to implement. If for any reason you can't carry out the program, or can handle only a portion of it, tell your physician. There are probably workable alternatives.

HERBAL MEDICINE

Herbalists use the leaves, flowers, stems, berries, and roots—either whole or in extract form—of plants to prevent, relieve, and treat illness. From a "scientific" perspective, many herbal treatments are considered experimental. The reality is, however, that herbal medicine has a long and respected history that is inextricably intertwined with the evolution of modern medicine. Many familiar medications of the twentieth century were developed from ancient healing traditions that treated health problems with specific plants. Today, science has isolated the medicinal properties of a large number of botanicals, and their healing components have been extracted and analyzed, with the result that many of them are now synthesized in large laboratories for use in pharmaceutical preparations. For example, salicylic acid, a precursor of aspirin, was originally derived from white willow bark and the meadowsweet plant; cinchona bark is the source of malaria-fighting quinine; vincristine, used to treat certain types of cancer, comes from periwinkle; and the opium poppy yields morphine (the standard against which new pain relievers are still measured), codeine, and paregoric, a treatment for diarrhea. However, once scientific methods were developed to extract and synthesize the active ingredients in plants, pharmaceutical laboratories took over from providers of medicinal herbs as the producers of drugs, and the paths of conventional medicine and herbal medicine began to diverge.

After decades of falling out of favor, herbal medicine has been undergoing a dramatic revival in recent years. Today, herbal products are available almost everywhere you turn. If you are interested in trying herbal medicine, it is important to understand that the quality of these products can vary greatly because there is a natural amount of variability in the active compounds that plants contain. Fortunately, there are now modern techniques that are being used to process herbal products. These manufacturing steps are as elaborate as those used to manufacture pharmaceutical products—sometimes, in fact, even more elaborate. Applying the principles of pharmaceutical manufacturing is done for good reason. Over the past forty-plus years, scientists have worked to identify active ingredients and substances termed *marker compounds* in herbs. Identifying active ingredients and/or marker compounds permits supplement producers to guarantee that their herbal preparations have a known percentage of active constituents and a known dosage. This process is called *standardization*. Standardized extracts are the most advanced form of herbal therapy available today. By being an informed consumer and knowing what to look for, you can be sure that you're getting what you pay for with herbal remedies. Read the label of any herbal product carefully before you buy it. Look for the following information:

- The name of the compound the standardization is based on.

- The percentage of that compound the extract contains.

- The extract ratio (for example, 50:1, 4:1, or whatever).

- The weight of each capsule or tablet.

- The number of capsules, tablets, or ounces per bottle.

- The recommended daily dosage (in therapeutic levels).

- The expiration date and product code (for tracking purposes).

- The manufacturer's name, address, telephone number, and/or Web site (so that you can contact the company for further information about the product).

A reputable company should also screen the product for the presence of pesticides, heavy metals, parasites, and fungal contamination, and determine the stability and consistency of the finished product.

Herbal treatment is useful for both acute and chronic conditions. It is also valuable in maintaining health and preventing illness. However, herbal medicines are not like pharmaceutical drugs. Herbal preparations work gently and take time to act. When you use an herbal preparation, begin with a small amount and watch closely for signs that symptoms are easing. Pay attention to how the preparation makes you feel. Also, while natural herbal preparations are generally well tolerated and are readily available without prescription in health food stores, drugstores, and other outlets, it is important to be aware that they *are* medicines, and they can have powerful effects. Also, as with any substance you ingest, it is possible to have a sensitivity to a particular herb that causes an unpleasant reaction such as a headache, an upset stomach, or a rash. Use your common sense, follow the manufacturer's directions, and, if you have questions or problems, seek the advice of a qualified health-care professional.

There is no formal licensing for herbalists, but it is possible to find professionals who practice herbal medicine, as well as other types of practitioners who prescribe herbs, including naturopaths, some chiropractors, and practitioners of traditional Chinese medicine, among others.

HOMEOPATHY

Homeopathy is a system of treatment, founded by German physician Samuel Hahnemann (1755–1843), that uses minute amounts of plant, mineral, and animal substances to stimulate the defensive systems of the body in a very subtle way. It has long been widely used in Europe, and its popularity in the United States is growing. The theoretical and empirical basis of homeopathy is a concept called the Law of Similars, often summarized as "like cures like." Perhaps more than anything else, what distinguishes the practice of homeopathy from other approaches to medicine is that instead of focusing on the specific causes of disease (such as viruses and bacteria), it focuses on the specifics of the *symptoms* of disease, *as they are experienced by the individual patient.* It is a systematic and precise form of natural medicine that addresses both physical and emotional symptoms and recognizes that each person is unique and will have an individual disease pattern. For example, you and another family member may have a cold caused by the same virus, yet one of you feels headachy, congested, and exhausted, while the other has a sore throat and a runny nose and feels restless. Homeopathic treatment takes account of such individual differences. The remedies stimulate the body's vital force and enhance its ability to heal itself in ways that are not scientifically understood. This fact is sometimes used as a basis for criticizing the practice. However, even today's most technologically advanced medical detectives do not really understand the ways in which body and mind work together. A complex interrelationship between immune factors and regenerative biological systems, the essential life force locked within body and mind remains a mystery. As best as we can explain it, homeopathic remedies work by "turning on a switch" that affects both body and mind. Homeopathic compounds somehow send a healing and normalizing message throughout the body. They spark unbalanced internal systems so that they are better able to perform their functions.

Many different types of health-care professionals incorporate homeopathy into their practice, among them medical doctors, naturopathic physicians, acupuncturists, herbalists, chiropractors, nurse practitioners, and physician assistants. Also, many books are available that can help you to try homeopathy on your own. (Unlike some other forms of health care, if you choose the "wrong" homeopathic treatment, it will not help, but it will not do any harm.)

BACH FLOWER REMEDIES

An offshoot of homeopathy is Bach flower therapy. This therapy involves the use of emotion-balancing flower preparations developed by Dr. Edward Bach (1897–1936). This approach is based on the belief that physical problems are root manifestations of emotional imbalances that can be addressed by dilute essences of plants known as Bach Flower Remedies. Unlike chemical mood-altering drugs, the flower remedies are gentle and easy to use, and can have remarkable emotional- and mental-balancing effects. Because they act quite gently, you can use them whenever you think they may help.

A variety of health-care practitioners can discuss the use of the flower remedies with you and help you to choose one or more that may be helpful. There are also books that can offer guidance. However, because the flower remedies are so benign, you can also try them quite safely on your own. Follow the instructions on the product label.

ACUPUNCTURE AND ACUPRESSURE

Acupressure is a gentle, noninvasive form of the ancient Chinese practice of acupuncture. In *acupuncture,* thin needles are inserted into the body at specific points along lines called meridians. In *acupressure,* thumb or finger pressure is applied at these same points, but the body is not punctured. In both practices, the aim is to effect beneficial changes and achieve harmony within the body's systems and structure. Both are based on the traditional Chinese medical philosophy, which views health in terms of a balance of vital energy, or *chi,* within the body. Each bodily organ must have the right amount of *chi* to function. Too much or too little *chi* causes an unbalance, resulting in illness or disease. *Chi* flows through all things, enters and passes through the body, creating harmony or disharmony. The goal of acupuncture and acupressure is to normalize the body's energies. *Chi* can be tapped at the meridians. Activating one key point sets up a predictable reaction in another area. By tonifying (increasing energy in) a specific area, the yin/yang balance is treated. Moving an excess of *chi* from one area and directing it to another, weaker area, corrects the yin/yang balance.

There are professionally trained and college-educated acupressurists, just as there are acupuncturists. Some massage therapists also utilize acupressure. It is also possible to experiment with it on your own, at home, with the help of a good book.

DIET AND NUTRITIONAL SUPPLEMENTS

One of the major changes in our understanding of health and disease in the past several decades is in the level of importance accorded to the role of diet. Certain foods also can be used medicinally for shorter-term problems—think of prunes for constipation, chicken soup for colds and flu, or a cup of strong coffee for migraine.

There was a time when conventional medical doctors were unlikely to say much, if anything, about diet to their patients. No more. Now health practitioners of virtually every type routinely include dietary advice in their treatment recommendations. Some use dietary approaches as a primary intervention, both preventively and in the short term, as well.

BASIC DIETARY GOALS

The Senate Select Committee on Nutrition and Human Services has developed a number of recommendations for ways Americans can improve their health through better nutrition. The following are the top five:

1. Increase your intake of fresh vegetables and whole grains.

2. Decrease your intake of refined and processed sugars.

3. Decrease your total fat consumption, and make sure the majority of fats you eat are healthy fats, such as those in olive oil and flaxseed oil.

4. Decrease your consumption of cholesterol.

5. Limit your salt intake.

We would add two others: Whenever possible, choose organic foods that are minimally processed (if at all) and free of artificial colors, flavors, and other additives; and don't overeat.

Recommendations for the use of nutritional supplements have been expanding; even the American Medical Association now recommends that everyone take a good multivitamin and multimineral supplement daily. There is a tremendous variety of nutritional supplements on the market, from the basic vitamins and minerals to more exotic-seeming compounds. Used correctly, supplements can provide long-term dietary "insurance" or short-term support to help your body heal from a particular illness or injury. For advice on diet and supplementation, a dietary counselor can be an excellent resource. There are many different kinds of professionals, with varied educational backgrounds and philosophies, who can recommend dietary programs and nutritional supplements. Registered dietitians, nutritionists, naturopathic physicians, chiropractors, medical doctors, and nurses—to name only a few—may all practice nutritional medicine. When interviewing a nutritional counselor, whether the person is a medical doctor or a macrobiotic counselor, find out about his or her educational background, work experience, and nutritional philosophy.

More detailed information about each of the healing approaches mentioned here, plus several others, as well as information about specific disorders and suggestions for how to utilize a complementary approach to health care to treat them, can be found in *Smart Medicine for a Healthier Child* (Avery/Penguin, 2003) and/or *Smart Medicine for Healthier Living* (Avery, 1999).

THE SMART MEDICINE CABINET

Every home should have a well-stocked home health kit. A good home health kit includes not only the bare essentials for dealing with emergencies, such as bandages, tweezers, and hydrogen peroxide, but also the basic medicines—conventional, herbal, homeopathic, and others—that are used over and over again for common illnesses. Your home health kit should be stored in a location that is convenient, but securely locked away from or out of the reach of children, and you should check it at least every three months or so to replace any products that have passed their expiration dates or that have been used up.

Begin putting your home health kit together now, so that the right treatments and remedies will be close at hand when you need them. Use the checklist that follows as a guide to some of the most important elements for a variety of different treatment approaches.

BARE ESSENTIALS

- Ace bandage
- Adhesive bandages (Band-Aids)
- Antibiotic topical
- Bulb syringe
- Hot-water bottle
- Ice bag
- Prescription insect bite kit containing adrenaline (such as Ana-Kit or EpiPen) if you or another family member has severe allergic reactions, whether to particular foods or to insect bites or stings
- Rescue Remedy Tincture
- Rubbing alcohol, hydrogen peroxide, or witch hazel, for disinfecting wounds and sterilizing needle and tweezers
- Scissors with rounded tips
- Sling and safety pins
- Sterile gauze pads and adhesive tape
- Sterile razor blade
- Sterilized needle
- Syrup of ipecac
  Caution: Syrup of ipecac should not be used except at the direction of a doctor or poison control center.
- Thermometer
- Tweezers

CONVENTIONAL MEDICATIONS

- Acetaminophen (Tylenol or the equivalent) or ibuprofen (Advil, Motrin, or the equivalent)

- An antihistamine (such as Benadryl or Chlor-Trimeton)

- An antiseptic ointment (such as bacitracin or Betadine)

- A decongestant (such as Sudafed)

- Emetrol syrup

- Milk of magnesia

- Pepto-Bismol

HERBAL MEDICINES

- Aloe vera gel

- Calendula cream

- Chamomile tea or extract

- Echinacea and goldenseal liquid combination formula

- Echinacea tincture

- Flaxseed tea

- Garlic, in capsules or fresh

- Ginger root, in capsules or fresh

- Licorice root extract

- Peppermint tea or extract

- Slippery elm powder

- Umeboshi plum paste

- Yin qiao tincture (liquid extract)

HOMEOPATHIC REMEDIES

- *Aconite*

- *Apis mellifica*

- *Arnica* ointment

- *Arnica*

- *Arsenicum album*

- *Belladonna*

- *Bryonia*

- *Calcarea carbonica*

- *Cantharis*

- *Carbo vegetabilis*

- *Chamomilla*

- *Ferrum phosphoricum*

- *Gelsemium*

- *Hepar sulphuris*

- *Hydrastis*

- *Hypericum* ointment

- *Hypericum*

- *Kali bichromicum*

- *Kali muriaticum*

- *Ledum*

- *Lycopodium*

- *Magnesia phosphorica*

- *Mercurius dulcis*

- *Mercurius solubilis*

- *Nux vomica*

- *Pulsatilla*

- *Rhus toxicodendron*

- *Ruta graveolens*

- *Sulphur*

- *Thuja*

- *Urtica urens* ointment

- *Urtica urens*

BACH FLOWER REMEDIES

- Rescue Remedy

NUTRITIONAL SUPPLEMENTS

- Calcium and magnesium combination formula (liquid or capsule)

- Vitamin-B complex liquid

- Vitamin C with bioflavonoids

- Zinc lozenges

MISCELLANEOUS

- Apple or grape juice, or applesauce, to mix with herbs or crushed tablets for anyone, such as a young child, who has trouble swallowing pills or capsules

- Eyedropper or needleless syringe to administer liquid medicines

- Honey, barley, malt, or rice bran syrup

In addition, the following are a number of important preventive measures you can take to prevent accidents, injuries, and other health problems:

- Post emergency telephone numbers near every telephone in your home. This can save precious time in any emergency. We urge you to take this precaution now, while you are thinking about it. If there is no 911 emergency service in your area, these numbers should include that of your local hospital for ambulance/paramedic service. Also post numbers for your local fire department, poison control center, police, and your doctor(s) and dentist. If you can program your telephone with numbers for automatic dialing, enter these emergency numbers into the phone as well, and label the appropriate keys clearly. Some telephones come with keys already labeled for police, fire, and other emergency numbers, which makes this even easier. However, you should not consider this a substitute for keeping emergency numbers on hand in written form. It is possible for programmed numbers to be erased accidentally, so you should still keep a list of emergency telephone numbers in a convenient location.

- Make sure that every room in your home has a working smoke detector and carbon monoxide detector. If detectors are wired in, it's a good idea to have a battery-operated backup in case of loss of electricity. Check and replace batteries as required.

- Set the temperature for the hot-water heater in your home no higher than 120°F. It takes only five seconds for 140°F water to cause a severe third-degree burn, but it takes a full three minutes to get a third-degree burn from 120°F water. Those extra minutes may provide enough time for you to prevent a nasty scald.

- Learn and practice safe food-handling and storage methods. Never store any potentially harmful object in food jars or food-storage containers.

- Keep a working fire extinguisher in a handy location near the stove (but out of the reach of children).

- Store all medicines and supplements in a cool, dry place—not in the bathroom medicine cabinet—and out of the reach of children. Do not take any medication that was prescribed for someone else, even if you have symptoms identical to those it was meant to treat. Throw away any medication that has passed its expiration date.

- Whether you are the driver or a passenger, always wear your seat belt when in a car. If you have young children, buckle them up securely in an approved safety restraint. *Never* drink and drive.

- Wear appropriate protective gear when engaging in sports activities. A helmet should be worn for bicycling, horseback riding, skiing, skateboarding, and Rollerblading. Goggles are useful for protecting your eyes from chlorine and other chemicals while swimming. Other types of protective gear that may be appropriate include knee pads, elbow pads, shin guards, mouth guards, and padded gloves.

- Learn to swim and learn water safety. When boating or engaging in sports such as water-skiing, wear a life jacket.

- Do not play with fireworks. Most states prohibit the sale of fireworks to individuals, but people still manage to obtain them. Every year, people suffer severe burns—or worse—from accidents connected with fireworks.

- Learn first aid and cardiopulmonary resuscitation (CPR). The Red Cross offers courses in these subjects, as do many hospitals. The important thing is to learn these procedures *before* you need to use them. If you have children, make sure any course you take includes a thorough grounding in infant and child CPR, and take a refresher course every year.

- Choose and empower surrogates who can act in your stead in an emergency if need be. Designate adults you trust—perhaps relatives, perhaps good friends—to make decisions in any emergency. Give your surrogates written permission to act for you, such as a limited power of attorney. Your surrogates should keep this important document where it can be found easily if they must respond to an emergency.

- If you or another member of your family has a special medical problem, obtain a Medic Alert bracelet to ensure that you will receive the right care if something happens away from home. If you are allergic to penicillin or other medication, sulfites, or bee stings, for example, this will enable you to receive prompt and appropriate treatment for an allergic reaction. Without a Medic Alert bracelet, a person with diabetes who is suffering from a low blood sugar reaction may be misdiagnosed as being intoxicated and fail to receive necessary treatment. Medic Alert information is especially important for a person who may not be able to communicate well or who has a disorder that can cause the loss of consciousness.

Not all accidents can be prevented, of course, but taking basic commonsense precautions such as those above and being prepared to deal with emergencies if they arise can save you from frantic searching and scrambling. This means faster treatment, as well as a less anxiety-filled experience, which in turn contributes to health and healing.

A GUIDE TO COMMON SYMPTOMS

The guide below lists some of the more common symptoms people experience, together with possible causes. Although you may be experiencing one or some of the symptoms listed here, you may or may not have any of the illnesses mentioned. Disorders are listed here because they *can* cause the particular symptom, and they are listed in alphabetical order, not in order of the likelihood of occurrence. This chart is not meant to substitute for the advice of a qualified health-care provider. Always consult with your doctor or other practitioner for a professional diagnosis.

Symptom	Possible Causes
Abdominal pain	Anxiety, appendicitis, candida infection, celiac disease, cirrhosis, constipation, Crohn's disease, diarrhea, diverticular disease, drug reaction or withdrawal, endometriosis, fibroids, food allergies, food poisoning, gallbladder problems, gas, hepatitis, hiatal hernia, indigestion, intestinal obstruction, intestinal parasites, irritable bowel syndrome, kidney disease, kidney stones, menstrual problems, motion sickness, nausea, pelvic inflammatory disease, peptic ulcer, premenstrual syndrome, urinary tract infection
Anal itching	Candida infection, contact allergy, gonorrhea, hemorrhoids, intestinal parasites, local irritation, rectal fissure, scabies, sexually transmitted disease, trichomoniasis
Appetite, increased	Anxiety, bulimia, depression, diabetes, drug abuse, drug reaction, hyperthyroidism, hypoglycemia, intestinal parasites, nicotine withdrawal, premenstrual syndrome
Appetite loss	Anemia, appendicitis, cancer, chronic fatigue syndrome, cirrhosis, constipation, Crohn's disease, depression, hepatitis, HIV disease, hyperthyroidism, kidney disease, secondary syphilis, tuberculosis, virtually any viral or bacterial infection
Backache	Kidney disease, kidney stones, low back pain, menstrual problems, muscle strain, premenstrual syndrome, prostatitis, stress, urinary tract infection
Bad breath	Diabetes, poor digestion, oral herpes, poor oral hygiene, postnasal drip, sinusitis, strep throat, tonsillitis, tooth decay
Bowel movement, painful	Constipation, Crohn's disease, hemorrhoids, irritable bowel syndrome, rectal fissure/tear
Breast pain/tenderness	Cancer, fibrocystic breast disease, hormonal fluctuations, premenstrual syndrome
Breathing difficulty/ shortness of breath	Anaphylactic shock, anemia, acute anxiety, asthma, cardiovascular disease, inhaled foreign object (choking), emphysema, hyperthyroidism, pneumonia, shock

Symptom	Possible Causes
Chest pain/discomfort	Acid reflux, acute anxiety, candida infection, cardiovascular disease, hiatal hernia, pneumonia
Concentrating, difficulty	Anxiety, chronic fatigue syndrome, concussion, drug abuse/withdrawal, drug reaction, nutritional deficiencies
Consciousness, loss of	Anaphylactic shock, concussion, drug abuse, drug reaction/withdrawal, meningitis, seizure, shock, stroke
Cough	Acid reflux, allergies, bronchitis, candida infection, common cold, flu, food allergy, hay fever, inhaled irritant, pneumonia, sore throat, stress, tuberculosis, viral or bacterial infection
Diarrhea	Anatomical deformity, candida infection, celiac disease, colitis, Crohn's disease, diverticular disease, drug reaction/withdrawal, fatigue, food allergy/sensitivity, food poisoning, hepatitis, HIV disease, intestinal parasites, irritable bowel syndrome, pancreatitis, virtually any viral, bacterial, fungal, or parasitic infection
Dizziness	Anemia, anxiety, cardiovascular disease, concussion, diabetic insulin reaction, drug abuse/withdrawal, drug reaction, eating disorders, fever, fibromyalgia, high blood pressure, hormonal fluctuations, hypoglycemia, Ménière's disease, motion sickness, multiple sclerosis, shock, stroke, temporomandibular joint syndrome
Earache	Common cold, ear infection, Ménière's disease, mumps, sinusitis, temporomandibular joint syndrome
Eating, difficulty	Cancer, canker sores, dry mouth, HIV disease, thrush
Eye inflammation/ watering/itching	Allergies, blepharitis, chalazion, common cold, conjunctivitis, contact-lens problems, corneal abrasion, food allergies, hay fever, onset of measles, stye
Eye pain	Contact-lens problems, dry eyes, eyestrain, acute glaucoma, uveitis
Fatigue/weakness	Anemia, anxiety, cancer, candida infection, cardiovascular disease, chronic fatigue syndrome, cirrhosis, Crohn's disease, depression, diabetes, drug reaction, eating disorder, flu, HIV disease, hyperthyroidism, hypoglycemia, hypothyroidism, insufficient sleep, intestinal parasites, lupus, Lyme or other tickborne disease, menopause, menstrual problems, mononucleosis, multiple sclerosis, poor nutrition, premenstrual syndrome, seizure, shock, sleep apnea, stress, stroke, virtually any viral or bacterial infection
Fever	Certain types of cancer, Crohn's disease, dehydration, diverticulitis, drug reaction/withdrawal, flu, inflamed gallbladder, heatstroke, hepatitis, HIV disease, kidney disease, lupus, meningitis, pelvic inflammatory disease, pneumonia, prostatitis, sinusitis, secondary syphilis, tuberculosis, virtually any viral or bacterial infection
Fluid retention/bloating/ swelling	Allergies, candida infection, cardiovascular disease, celiac disease, cirrhosis, food allergies, hormonal fluctuations, kidney disease, lymphedema, premenstrual syndrome
Hair loss	Drug reaction, heredity, hormonal fluctuations, lupus, nutritional deficiencies, physical trauma, ringworm, shingles, stress, secondary syphilis, thyroid disorders, tuberculosis
Headache	Anemia, cancer (brain tumor), chronic fatigue syndrome, concussion, diabetic insulin reaction, drug reaction/withdrawal, eyestrain, fibromyalgia, food allergies, acute glaucoma, high blood pressure, hormonal imbalance, hypoglycemia, Lyme disease, meningitis, menopause, migraine, mononucleosis, mumps, premenstrual syndrome, sinusitis, stress, stroke, temporomandibular joint syndrome, uveitis
Hearing loss/disturbance	Ear infection, Ménière's disease, stroke, temporomandibular joint syndrome, tinnitus
Heartbeat, irregular/heart palpitations	Anaphylactic shock, anemia, anorexia nervosa, anxiety, bulimia, cardiovascular disease, drug abuse/withdrawal, drug reaction, fibromyalgia, hyperthyroidism, Lyme disease, menopause, shock, stress
Irritability/agitation/restlessness	Alcoholism, Alzheimer's disease, onset of anaphylactic shock, anxiety, diabetes, drug abuse, drug reaction/withdrawal, hyperthyroidism, hypoglycemia, meningitis, menopause, premenstrual syndrome, shock, stress

Symptom	Possible Causes
Jaw pain	Injury, mumps, sinusitis, temporomandibular joint syndrome, tetanus, tooth decay
Joint pain	Arthritis, bunion, bursitis, candida infection, chronic fatigue syndrome, fibromyalgia, gout, intestinal parasites, lupus, Lyme or other tickborne disease, rheumatic fever, sprain, secondary syphilis
Light sensitivity	Blepharitis, concussion, corneal abrasion, drug abuse/ withdrawal, drug reaction, glaucoma, hyperthyroidism, onset of measles, onset of migraine, photophobia, uveitis
Lymph nodes, enlarged	Chronic fatigue syndrome, genital herpes, HIV disease, Lyme or other tickborne disease, mononucleosis, virtually any viral or bacterial infection
Malaise (general bodywide discomfort)	Anxiety, chronic fatigue syndrome, depression, fever, fibromyalgia, food poisoning, hepatitis, intestinal parasites, lupus, mononucleosis, virtually any viral or bacterial infection
Memory lapses	Alcoholism, allergies, Alzheimer's disease, anxiety, systemic candidiasis, chronic fatigue syndrome, concussion, drug abuse, drug reaction, fibromyalgia, inattention, stress
Menstrual bleeding, abnormal/heavy	Cancer, endometriosis, fibroids, hypothyroidism, pelvic inflammatory disease
Menstrual bleeding, absent/scant	Cancer, eating disorders, hyperthyroidism, menopause, severe weight loss, stress
Mood/personality changes	Alcoholism, Alzheimer's disease, anxiety, chronic fatigue syndrome, chronic pain, depression, drug abuse/withdrawal, drug reaction, fibromyalgia, hormonal fluctuations, hypoglycemia, manic-depressive disorder, menopause, multiple sclerosis, premenstrual syndrome, stress
Mouth sores	Canker sores, oral herpes, HIV disease, onset of measles, nutritional deficiencies, thrush
Muscle aches and pains	Candida infection, chronic fatigue syndrome, fibromyalgia, hypothyroidism, Lyme or other tickborne disease, menopause, multiple sclerosis, muscle strain, overexertion, restless legs syndrome, sprain, tendinitis, virtually any viral or bacterial infection
Muscle rigidity	Multiple sclerosis, Parkinson's disease, seizure, tetanus
Nose, runny and/or stuffy	Allergies, bronchitis, candida infection, common cold, drug abuse, drug reaction/withdrawal, food allergies, hay fever, sinusitis
Numbness/tingling sensations	Anxiety, candida infection, carpal tunnel syndrome, concussion, drug reaction, hypothyroidism, multiple sclerosis, Raynaud's phenomenon, restless legs syndrome, seizure, stroke
Sex drive, altered	Alcoholism, anxiety, depression, drug abuse, drug reaction, menopause, chronic pain, premenstrual syndrome, stress
Sexual intercourse, painful	Chlamydia, endometriosis, fibroids, pelvic inflammatory disease, trichomoniasis, vaginitis
Skin rash, lesions, or bumps	Acne, allergies, athlete's foot, boil, bruises, candida infection, chickenpox, dandruff, dermatitis, eczema, heat rash, herpes, insect bites, intestinal parasites, lupus, Lyme or other tickborne disease, measles, poison ivy, psoriasis, ringworm, rosacea, scabies, seborrhea, shingles, skin cancer, sunburn, syphilis, varicose veins, warts
Sleep difficulties	Anemia, anxiety, chronic fatigue syndrome, chronic pain, depression, drug abuse/withdrawal, drug reaction, fibromyalgia, hyperthyroidism, irregular schedule, jet lag, menopause, restless legs syndrome, sleep apnea, snoring, stress
Stools, bloody/rectal bleeding	Cancer, colitis, Crohn's disease, diverticular disease, hemorrhoids, rectal tear/fissure
Sweating, excessive	Onset of anaphylactic shock, acute anxiety, cardiovascular disease, drug abuse/withdrawal, drug reaction, diabetic insulin reaction, heat exhaustion, high blood pressure, HIV disease, hyperthyroidism, hypoglycemia, overexertion, shock
Testicular pain	Cancer, epididymitis, mumps

Symptom	Possible Causes
Thirst, excessive	Dehydration, diabetes, drug reaction/withdrawal
Tremors	Anxiety, drug abuse/withdrawal, drug reaction, hyperthyroidism, hypoglycemia, Parkinson's disease, seizure, stress, stroke
Urination, difficult/painful	Chlamydia, fibroids, gonorrhea, genital herpes, prostate disorders, trichomoniasis, urinary tract infection, vaginitis
Urination, frequent	Diabetes, excessive fluid intake, kidney stones, enlarged prostate, urinary tract infection
Urine, bloody	Dehydration, hepatitis, kidney disease, kidney stones, prostate disorders, urinary tract infection
Vaginal/vulvar itching	Candida infection, chlamydia, local irritation, trichomoniasis, vaginitis
Vaginal discharge	Candida infection, chlamydia, fibroids, gonorrhea, pelvic inflammatory disease, trichomoniasis, vaginitis
Vision loss/disturbance	Cataracts, floaters, glaucoma, hypoglycemia, macular degeneration, onset of migraine or seizure, multiple sclerosis, photophobia, presbyopia, retinal disorders, stroke, uveitis
Vomiting	Anxiety, celiac disease, drug abuse/withdrawal, drug reaction, cirrhosis, food allergies, food poisoning, fatigue, hepatitis, HIV disease, kidney disease, Ménière's disease, migraine, motion sickness, overeating, poisoning, shock, stress, virtually any systemic viral or bacterial infection
Weight gain, unintended	Poor eating habits, hypothyroidism, slowed metabolism, premenstrual syndrome
Weight loss, unintended	Anorexia nervosa, anxiety, cancer, celiac disease, cirrhosis, Crohn's disease, depression, diabetes, drug abuse, poor eating habits, HIV disease, lupus, tuberculosis
Wheezing	Anaphylaxic shock, allergies, asthma, bronchitis, hay fever

PART TWO

CHILDREN'S GROWTH AND DEVELOPMENT RECORDS

YOUR CHILD AT BIRTH

ake this book with you to the hospital or birthing center, or keep it handy for the big event at home if you are planning a home birth, so that you can start recording important health information about your child as soon as possible after birth. Use the spaces that follow to record your baby's vital statistics and any procedures performed, problems encountered, or treatments administered, as well as any recommendations or observations from your health-care provider. There is also space for an imprint of your newborn's footprints and room for observations, thoughts, and reflections from you. And congratulations!

BIRTH DATA

Baby's name: _____

Baby's exact date and time of birth: _____

Weight: _____ Length: _____ Head circumference: _____

Apgar score: 1 _____ 2 _____

The Apgar score is an evaluation of your infant's overall condition, based on five key characteristics: color, respiration, heart rate, muscle tone, and reflexes.

Characteristic	0 Points	1 Point	2 Points
Color	Blue, pale	Body pink, extremities blue	Body completely pink
Respiratory Effort	Absent	Slow, irregular, weak cry	Strong cry
Heart Rate	Absent	Less than 100 beats per minute	More than 100 beats per minute
Muscle Tone	Limp	Some flexing of extremities	Active motion
Reflexes	Absent	Grimace, some motion	Cry

Your baby's first Apgar score, taken a minute after birth, is an indication of how your newborn came through labor and delivery, as well as how the child is likely to fare in the postpartum period. A score of 8 to 10 means that a newborn's condition is good. A low rating alerts the medical staff that the child needs extra care. After five minutes has passed, a second Apgar rating is given. This additional test will show the doctor how your newborn is adjusting to life outside the womb. Ask your doctor or nurse for the Apgar scores your baby was given and record them in the blanks above.

POST-BIRTH PROCEDURES

There are a number of procedures that may be performed on a baby in the hours or days following birth. Record the procedures performed on your baby in the following table. Note that not all of these procedures may be deemed necessary for your child; conversely, you may need to add others not already listed here if they are recommended. If you have concerns about any of these procedures, discuss this with your doctor beforehand and come to an agreement as to what will and will not be done—and get a signed agreement to this effect—to avoid misunderstandings amid the excitement (and exhaustion) following birth.

Procedure	Performed?
Antibiotic ointment or silver nitrate solution instilled in the eyes	
Silver nitrate solution drops in the eyes	
Vitamin K injection administered	
Complete physical examination (including measurement and inspection of the cardiorespiratory system, musculoskeletal system, nervous system, skin, head, eyes, ears, mouth, abdomen, and genitalia)	
Initial bath	
Circumcision	

SCREENING TESTS

A number of screening tests are routinely performed on newborns born in hospitals. The exact tests done (some of which may be required by law) may vary from state to state, and tests other than the routine ones may be added if your child is considered to be at risk for a particular disorder. Use the following table to record which screening tests have been done on your child and what the results were.

Screening Test	Result
Biotinidase deficiency (BIO), also known as multiple carboxylase deficiency (MCD), carboxylase deficiency multiple, and holocarboxylase synthetase deficiency. This is a congenital disorder that results from impaired activity of three enzymes that depend on the B vitamin biotin, caused by a defect in cellular transport or metabolism of biotin. It can lead to acidosis (excessively acidic blood and tissues), seizures, developmental delays, skin rashes, and hearing loss. These problems can be prevented if an affected child is treated with biotin.	
Congenital adrenal hyperplasia (CAH). This is a condition caused by a genetic defect in the adrenal glands that renders them unable to produce certain vital hormones known as corticosteroids. This makes it harder for the body to cope with the physical effects of stress from all sources. CAH is treated with medication to replace the missing hormones.	
Congenital hypothyroidism (CH). This is a disorder caused by insufficient production of thyroid hormone as a result of a malfunctioning thyroid gland. It can lead to impaired growth and other problems. CH is treated with medication to replace the missing hormone.	
Galactosemia (GAL). This is a genetic disorder that results from a lack of one of the enzymes necessary to break down galactose, a form of monosaccharide (simple sugar) that is a component of many polysaccharide (complex sugar) molecules, most importantly lactose (milk sugar). This causes galactose to build up to unhealthy levels in the blood, and can lead to cataracts, liver damage, neurological damage, developmental delays, and even death. These problems can be avoided by giving an affected child a special formula instead of milk. People with galactosemia must follow a restricted diet for life to avoid problems.	
Homocystinuria (HCY). This is a condition that occurs if a person is unable to use methionine, an amino acid that is a component of many proteins found in food. If untreated, it can result in developmental delays, neurological damage, and, ultimately, death. Treatment with supplements of vitamin B_6 and/or a restricted low-protein diet can help to prevent these problems.	
Human immunodeficiency virus (HIV). This is the virus that causes AIDS. If a newborn tests positive for HIV, retesting will be recommended, as it is possible for the virus to become undetectable in the months after birth. The health of a mother of a child who tests positive for HIV will also need to be monitored. While there is no cure for HIV, there are drug treatments available that can improve longevity and quality of life for people who are infected.	
Maple syrup urine disease (MSUD). This is a genetic disorder that got its name because it makes an individual's urine smell like maple syrup. It is caused by the body's inability to utilize a number of amino acids, building blocks of proteins, and can result in seizures, developmental delays, and even death. It is treated with a special protein-restricted diet.	
Phenylketonuria (PKU). This is a congenital disorder caused by the inability to break down the amino acid phenylalanine. It can lead to developmental delays and other problems, but these consequences can be prevented by eliminating all sources of phenylalanine from a child's diet.	
Sickle cell disease (SCD). This is an inherited disorder characterized by a defect in hemoglobin, resulting in red blood cells that have an abnormal shape and cannot carry oxygen efficiently to the body's cells. This in turn can lead to frequent infections and other problems. It requires lifelong management and is often treated with antibiotics.	
Tandem mass spectrometry screening (MS/MS). This is a type of testing that is done to screen for a number of different metabolic problems.	
Other screening tests (list): _____ _____ _____ _____	

OTHER INFORMATION

Health problems encountered after birth, if any: _____

_____

_____

_____

_____

_____

Treatments administered: _____

_____

_____

_____

_____

_____

Additional observations/recommendations of health-care provider: _____

_____

_____

_____

_____

_____

YOUR BABY'S FOOTPRINTS

Shortly after your baby is born, your fingerprints and your newborn's footprints will be recorded for identification purposes. The nurse can also put your baby's foot-prints in this book in the space below.

YOUR OBSERVATIONS AND REFLECTIONS

CHILDREN'S HEIGHT AND WEIGHT CHARTS

The graphs on the pages that follow represent heights and weights for boys and girls aged two to twenty years, with lines showing the percentile of the population for different heights and weights. You can use these to chart your own child's height and weight, and see where he or she falls as compared with other American children. Keep in mind, though, that there is no "best" height or weight; every child is an individual. If you have concerns about your child's growth pattern, consult your health-care practitioner.

CDC GROWTH CHARTS: UNITED STATES

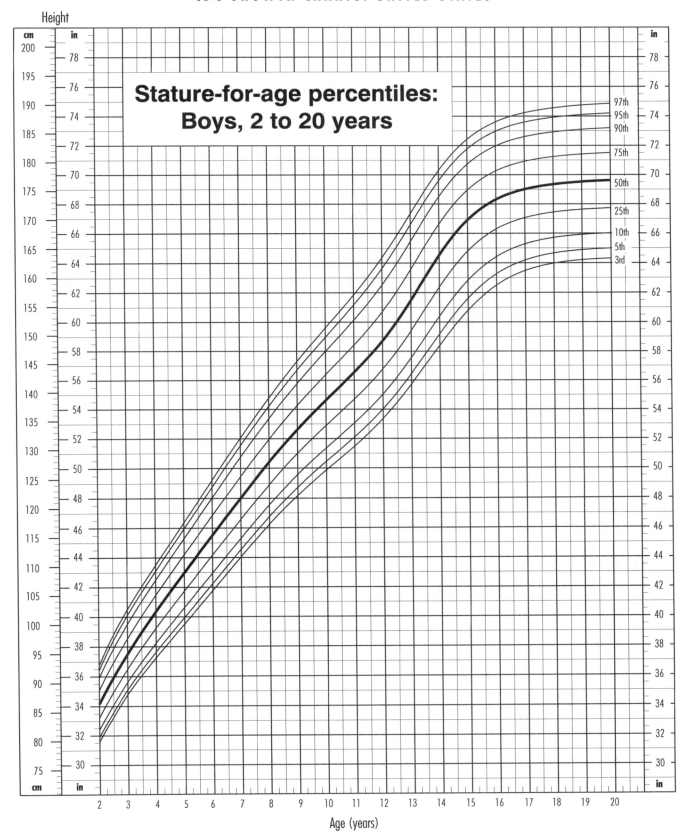

Height

**Stature-for-age percentiles:
Boys, 2 to 20 years**

Age (years)

CDC GROWTH CHARTS: UNITED STATES

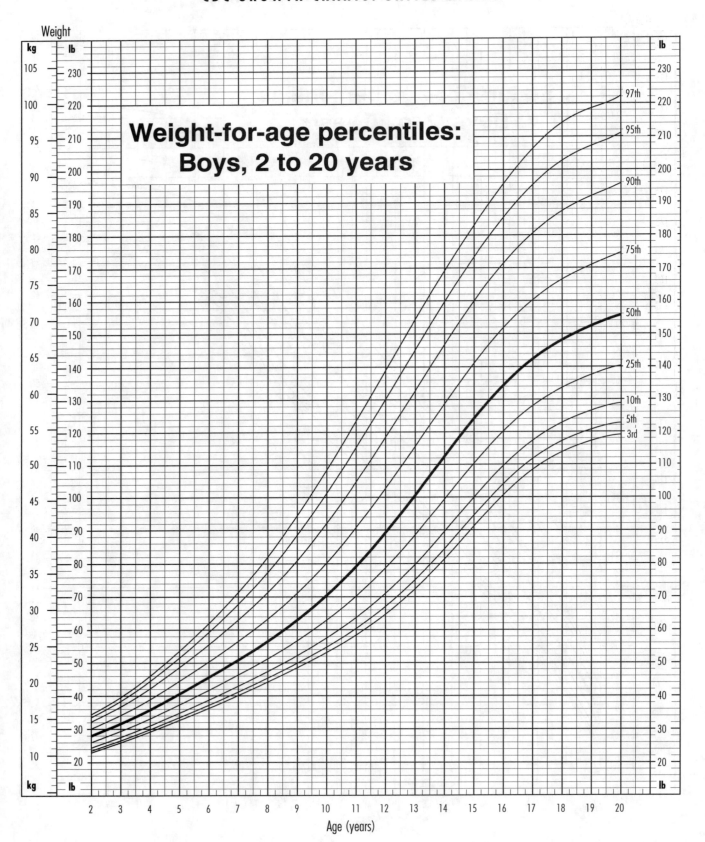

Weight

Weight-for-age percentiles: Boys, 2 to 20 years

Age (years)

CDC GROWTH CHARTS: UNITED STATES

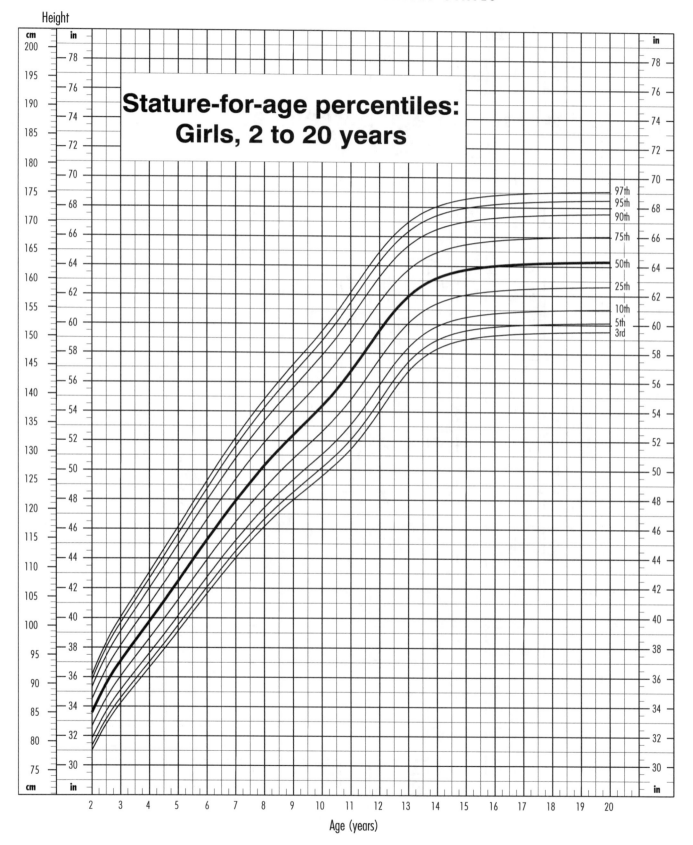

Height

**Stature-for-age percentiles:
Girls, 2 to 20 years**

Age (years)

CDC GROWTH CHARTS: UNITED STATES

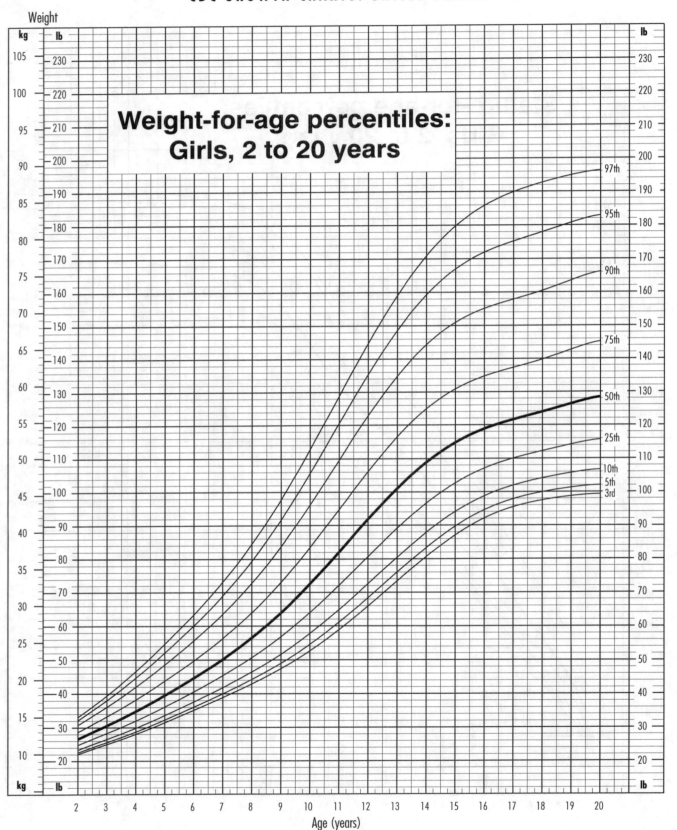

Weight-for-age percentiles: Girls, 2 to 20 years

DEVELOPMENTAL MILESTONES

Raising a child means encountering a series of "firsts." These are often exciting and rewarding. There may also come a time when information about a child's early developmental history may yield important clues for health-care providers. Use the table below to record some of the notable milestones in your baby's growth and development. And keep in mind that all children develop at their own pace. There is no one "normal" standard that applies to all children.

Milestone	Your Observations/ Date	Details
PHYSICAL DEVELOPMENT		
Baby smiles for the first time.		
Baby begins to hold his or her head up.		
Baby rolls over for the first time.		
Baby's first tooth erupts.		
Baby sits up unassisted.		
Baby starts crawling.		
Baby pulls him- or herself up into a standing position.		
Baby stands unassisted.		
Baby takes his or her first step.		
LANGUAGE DEVELOPMENT		
Baby starts vocalizing (other than crying!).		
Baby starts "babbling" in imitation of adult speech.		
Baby speaks his or her first recognizable word.		
Baby says his or her first simple sentence.		

DIET DIARY

When to introduce a baby to solid foods is a subject of some controversy. Some recommend starting solids at about six months of age; others say it is best for a baby to be breastfed exclusively for at least a year. Whenever you start feeding your baby solid foods, it is a good idea to introduce foods one at a time to determine how your baby responds to them. It is not uncommon for a baby to have an allergic reaction to a new food. Allergies can lead to obvious symptoms such as skin rashes and nasal congestion, but can also cause more subtle problems, including itchiness and stomachache. Use the pages that follow to record your child's reactions to the foods you introduce. You can use a similar system to record information about diet and symptoms for an individual of any age if you suspect food allergies.

Date	Time	Food/Amount Eaten	Responses

Date	Time	Food/Amount Eaten	Responses

Date	Time	Food/Amount Eaten	Responses

Date	Time	Food/Amount Eaten	Responses

Date	Time	Food/Amount Eaten	Responses

Date	Time	Food/Amount Eaten	Responses

Date	Time	Food/Amount Eaten	Responses

Date	Time	Food/Amount Eaten	Responses

Date	Time	Food/Amount Eaten	Responses

Date	Time	Food/Amount Eaten	Responses

IMMUNIZATION RECORD

An immunization, or vaccination, is an injection of weakened or killed bacteria, viruses, or, in some cases, deactivated toxins that is given to protect against or reduce the effects of certain infectious diseases. When your child receives an injection of, for example, a small amount of tetanus toxoid, her immune system produces antibodies to fight this foreign substance. Should your child later be exposed to tetanus, her body's defense system will remember and rapidly form antibodies against the bacteria, thus preventing the disease from gaining a hold within the body.

The following vaccinations are among those most commonly recommended for children.

- DPT, or diphtheria/pertussis/tetanus, is designed to protect against three different diseases: diphtheria, a rare but potentially fatal disease that affects the upper respiratory tract, the heart, and kidneys; pertussis, or whooping cough, a disease that is particularly dangerous for children under one year of age and can lead to pneumonia, seizures, and other complications; and tetanus, a potentially deadly infection of the central nervous system.

- DT, or diphtheria/tetanus, is an alternative to DPT, without the pertussis vaccine. It is designed to protect against diphtheria and tetanus only.

- *Hemophilus influenzae* (*H. flu.*) meningitis type B vaccine, or Hib vaccine, protects against a common bacterial infection that can lead to meningitis, a potentially fatal brain disease. A combination DPT and Hib vaccine is available that reduces the number of injections a child must receive to be immunized against all of these diseases.

- The hepatitis B vaccine protects against one of the more serious forms of hepatitis, hepatitis B. This is an infection of the liver that, while not highly contagious, can lead to chronic liver disease or even liver cancer.

- MMR, or measles/mumps/rubella, also works to prevent three different diseases: measles, a highly contagious viral disease characterized by fever and rash, whose danger lies in the possibility of such serious complications as pneumonia, strep infections, and encephalitis; mumps, a contagious viral disease that causes fever and swollen glands around the neck and throat (and, rarely, the testicles); and rubella, or German measles, a viral disease involving fever and a mild rash that causes relatively little discomfort to the affected child, but that can cause miscarriage, stillbirth, or birth defects if a woman is exposed to the virus during pregnancy.

· The polio vaccine is designed to protect against poliomyelitis, an acute viral infection that can lead to paralysis and death.

· Immunization against rubella may be recommended if your child is a girl between thirteen and sixteen years old who has not received the MMR vaccine (see above) or had German measles.

· The tetanus toxoid vaccine protects against tetanus, an infection of the central nervous system that can be fatal. It is usually given to children in the form of a DPT or DT immunization (see above), but it can be administered individually.

· Varicella is designed to protect against the virus that causes chickenpox. It is given as a single dose to children between the ages of twelve months and thirteen years that have never had chickenpox. Children over age thirteen require an additional booster after the first dose.

Other immunizations or changes in the conventional immunization schedule may be recommended for special reasons, such as illness or travel. Some vaccinations are repeated at intervals to achieve immunity. Use the forms that follow to keep track of your children's immunization history and to serve as a reminder of when immunization status needs updating. Have your doctor sign it in the appropriate location in the right-hand column; that way, you will have ready proof of your child's immunization status for occasions when you need it, such as before your child starts school.

Child's name: _____   **Date of birth:** _____

Recommended Age	Vaccine	Date Administered	Doctor's Signature	Baby's Response
1–2 days	Hepatitis B[1]			
1–2 months	Hepatitis B[2]			
2 months	DPT or DT[1] Hemophilus B[1] Pneumococcus[1] Polio[1]			
4 months	DPT or DT[2] Hemophilus B[2] Pneumococcus[2] Polio[2]			
6 months	DPT or DT[3] Hemophilus B[3] Pneumococcus[3]			
6–18 months	Hepatitis B[3] Polio[3]			
12–15 months	Hemophilus B[1] MMR Pneumococcus			
12–18 months	Varicella			
15–18 months	DPT or DT			
4–6 years	DPT or DT MMR Polio			
11–12 years	DT			
13–16 years	Rubella[3]			
14–16 years	Tetanus			

1. May be given in combination with DPT.
2. U.S. Centers for Disease Control and Prevention recommends that a second dose of this vaccine be given before a child enters school; the American Academy of Pediatrics recommends that this be done later, when a child is entering middle or junior high school.
3. For girls only, this vaccine may be recommended if a child is unimmunized (that is, did not receive the MMR vaccine) and has not developed sufficient antibodies as a result of having the disease.

WELL-BABY VISITS

Your child's first encounter with a pediatrician or family physician is likely to come moments after birth. The doctor will perform a physical assessment of your new baby to be sure he or she is healthy. Following the initial assessment, it is wise to keep regular well-baby and then well-child visits. Your doctor will likely recommend an appropriate schedule. If an emerging health problem is discovered during a well-child examination, care and treatment can begin at the optimum moment. In addition, your doctor can reassure you about your child's physical growth and development, and offer guidance concerning cognitive and emotional growth and development. Use the forms on the pages that follow to record details of your child's well-baby visits.

Cord Care

The stump of a newborn's umbilical cord will fall off some time between one and three weeks after you take your baby home. In the meantime, remember the following about cord care:

- To keep the area dry and free of urine, fold your baby's diaper down.

- Until the cord has fallen off and the area has healed completely, give only sponge baths.

- While this small wound is healing, clean the stump and entire area with rubbing alcohol a few times each day. Using a cotton swab dipped in rubbing alcohol or calendula tincture, clean the stump, around the cord, at the base of the cord, and between the skin and the cord.

- The area may ooze and drip a small amount of blood for a few days after the stump has come off. The area will scab over. Don't pick at or remove the scab. Allow it to fall off naturally.

- During this entire period, watch for any signs of infection. If the area becomes red, swollen, oozes pus, or becomes tender, call your doctor.

Child's name:

Date of birth:

Well-baby visit number: Date:

Baby's age:

Practitioner consulted:

General Physical Examination:

Weight: pounds   ounces   Length/height: inches

Head circumference: inches   Other:

Developmental/behavioral evaluation:

Tests and screening procedures performed, if any:

Test (specify)

Result

Test (specify)

Result

Test (specify)

Result

Test (specify)

Result

Test (specify)

Result

Immunizations, if any:

Treatments administered, if any:

Practitioner's observations/recommendations/answers to questions:

Your child's responses to recommended measures:

Other observations:

Questions to ask doctor at the next visit:

Child's name: .... Date of birth: ....

Well-baby visit number: .... Date: .... Baby's age: ....

Practitioner consulted: ....

General Physical Examination: ....

Weight: .... pounds .... ounces .... Length/height: .... inches .... Head circumference: .... inches

Other: ....

....

Developmental/behavioral evaluation: ....

Tests and screening procedures performed, if any: ....

    Test (specify) ....

    Result ....

    Test (specify) ....

    Result ....

    Test (specify) ....

    Result ....

    Test (specify) ....

    Result ....

    Test (specify) ....

    Result ....

Immunizations, if any: ....

....

Treatments administered, if any: ....

....

....

Practitioner's observations/recommendations/answers to questions: ....

....

....

....

Your child's responses to recommended measures: ....

....

....

Other observations: ....

....

....

Questions to ask doctor at the next visit: ....

....

....

Child's name: .... Date of birth: ....

Well-baby visit number: .... Date: .... Baby's age: ....

Practitioner consulted: ....

General Physical Examination: ....

Weight: .... pounds .... ounces   Length/height: .... inches

Head circumference: .... inches   Other: ....

Your Baby's Reflexes

Babies are born with a number of reflexes, which function as important survival and protective devices. These reflexes include the following:

- The rooting reflex: When you touch a newborn's cheek, he or she will automatically turn his or her head in that direction and "root" around looking for mother's breast.

- The suckling reflex: This is the instinct to suck. A newborn baby may suck a thumb or a finger, or even try to stuff an entire tiny fist in his or her mouth.

- The swallowing reflex: When a newborn suckles, he or she instinctively swallows as needed. This was learned in the womb, where the developing baby swallowed and excreted amniotic fluid.

- The gag reflex and the cough reflex: If something gets in a newborn's mouth that shouldn't be there, he or she will gag to expel it. The gagging reflex helps protect against choking. The cough reflex helps your infant get rid of an accumulation of mucus.

Developmental/behavioral evaluation: ....

Tests and screening procedures performed, if any:

Test (specify) ....

Result ....

Test (specify) ....

Result ....

Test (specify) ....

Result ....

Test (specify) ....

Result ....

Test (specify) ....

Result ....

Immunizations, if any: ....

Treatments administered, if any: ....

Practitioner's observations/recommendations/answers to questions: ....

Your child's responses to recommended measures: ....

Other observations: ....

Questions to ask doctor at the next visit: ....

Child's name: .... Date of birth: ....

Well-baby visit number: .... Date: .... Baby's age: ....

Practitioner consulted: ....

General Physical Examination:

Weight: .... pounds .... ounces .... Length/height: .... inches ....

Head circumference: .... inches .... Other: ....

Developmental/behavioral evaluation: ....

Tests and screening procedures performed, if any:

    Test (specify) ....

    Result ....

    Test (specify) ....

    Result ....

    Test (specify) ....

    Result ....

    Test (specify) ....

    Result ....

    Test (specify) ....

    Result ....

Immunizations, if any: ....

Treatments administered, if any: ....

....

Practitioner's observations/recommendations/answers to questions: ....

....

....

Your child's responses to recommended measures: ....

....

....

Other observations: ....

....

Questions to ask doctor at the next visit: ....

....

....

- The grasp reflex: When you place a finger or two in a newborn's palm, he or she will respond with a firm, instinctive grip.

- The stepping reflex: When you hold a baby upright, supported under the arms, he or she will "step out" in a walking motion.

- The tonic neck reflex: This describes the typical "fencing position" a baby often assumes. A newborn may lie on his or her back, with the head turned to one side and the arm and leg on that side extended, while the other arm and leg are flexed. If the neck is rotated quickly, the baby will respond by extending the opposite arm and leg, while the previously extended limbs will flex.

- The Moro reflex: When a newborn is startled, he or she will typically thrust both arms out with a sudden, jerky motion, as if asking for a hug. This "parachute" helps to protect an infant in the event of a fall.

Child's name: .... Date of birth: ....

Well-baby visit number: .... Date: .... Baby's age: ....

Practitioner consulted: ....

General Physical Examination: ....

Weight: .... pounds .... ounces .... Length/height: .... inches .... Head circumference: .... inches

Other: ....

....

Developmental/behavioral evaluation: ....

Tests and screening procedures performed, if any: ....

    Test (specify) ....

    Result ....

    Test (specify) ....

    Result ....

    Test (specify) ....

    Result ....

    Test (specify) ....

    Result ....

    Test (specify) ....

    Result ....

Immunizations, if any: ....

....

Treatments administered, if any: ....

....

....

Practitioner's observations/recommendations/answers to questions: ....

....

....

....

Your child's responses to recommended measures: ....

....

....

Other observations: ....

....

....

Questions to ask doctor at the next visit: ....

....

....

Child's name: .... Date of birth: ....

Well-baby visit number: .... Date: .... Baby's age: ....

Practitioner consulted: ....

General Physical Examination: ....

Weight: .... pounds .... ounces .... Length/height: .... inches .... Head circumference: .... inches

Other: ....
....

Developmental/behavioral evaluation: ....

Tests and screening procedures performed, if any: ....

　　　Test (specify) ....

　　　Result ....

　　　Test (specify) ....

　　　Result ....

　　　Test (specify) ....

　　　Result ....

　　　Test (specify) ....

　　　Result ....

　　　Test (specify) ....

　　　Result ....

Immunizations, if any: ....
....

Treatments administered, if any: ....
....
....

Practitioner's observations/recommendations/answers to questions: ....
....
....
....

Your child's responses to recommended measures: ....
....
....

Other observations: ....
....

Questions to ask doctor at the next visit: ....
....
....

Child's name: .... Date of birth: ....

Well-baby visit number: .... Date: .... Baby's age: ....

Practitioner consulted: ....

General Physical Examination: ....

Weight: .... pounds .... ounces .... Length/height: .... inches

Head circumference: .... inches .... Other: ....

Babies' Height and Weight Development

Not all babies grow at the same rate, of course, but the following are some general ideas of the average baby's growth and weight gain:

- In the first few days after birth, babies lose 5 to 10 percent of their birth weight. This weight is gradually gained back over a period of two to three weeks.

- During the first three months of life, infants gain about two pounds each month.

- Between three months and one year of age, babies gain about one pound each month.

- On average, by the age of one year, babies are triple their weight and are 50 percent longer than they were at birth.

Developmental/behavioral evaluation: ....

Tests and screening procedures performed, if any:

Test (specify) ....

Result ....

Test (specify) ....

Result ....

Test (specify) ....

Result ....

Test (specify) ....

Result ....

Test (specify) ....

Result ....

Immunizations, if any: ....

Treatments administered, if any: ....

Practitioner's observations/recommendations/answers to questions: ....

Your child's responses to recommended measures: ....

Other observations: ....

Questions to ask doctor at the next visit: ....

Child's name: .... Date of birth: ....

Well-baby visit number: .... Date: .... Baby's age: ....

Practitioner consulted: ....

General Physical Examination: ....

Weight: .... pounds .... ounces Length/height: .... inches Head circumference: .... inches

Other: ....

Developmental/behavioral evaluation: ....

Tests and screening procedures performed, if any: ....

     Test (specify) ....

     Result ....

     Test (specify) ....

     Result ....

     Test (specify) ....

     Result ....

     Test (specify) ....

     Result ....

     Test (specify) ....

     Result ....

Immunizations, if any: ....

Treatments administered, if any: ....

Practitioner's observations/recommendations/answers to questions: ....

Your child's responses to recommended measures: ....

Other observations: ....

Questions to ask doctor at the next visit: ....

Child's name: .... Date of birth: ....

Well-baby visit number: .... Date: .... Baby's age: ....

Practitioner consulted: ....

General Physical Examination: ....

Weight: .... pounds .... ounces   Length/height: .... inches

Head circumference: .... inches   Other: ....

A Few Words about Sleep

Newborns usually spend about 80 percent of their resting/sleeping time in shallow sleep, and only about 20 percent of the time in deep sleep. When newborns seem to be sleeping, they are usually very close to awakening.

Some babies sleep easily. Others do not. Many babies (and parents) get their best sleep with the baby resting on the parent's chest or in the parents' bed with them. This position helps to satisfy a baby's deep need for round-the-clock attention or cuddling. Modern Western nations have the only cultures in the world with a taboo against babies sleeping with their parents. Resting or sleeping with your child in the crook of your arm will comfort your newborn, and can relax and soothe a sleepy, lonely toddler as well.

Sleeping in the prone (stomach-down) position may be a factor in sudden infant death syndrome (SIDS), especially when a baby lies on a very soft surface, such as sheepskin. This can cause a dangerous buildup of carbon dioxide in the blood, which may cause the baby to stop breathing. Doctors recommend that infants sleep either in a supine position (on their backs) or on their sides. After a feeding, it is best to keep a baby on his or her side, with the back supported by a pillow. If the baby should spit up in this position, the milk will drain out of his or her mouth and there will be no risk of choking.

Developmental/behavioral evaluation: ....

Tests and screening procedures performed, if any: ....

Test (specify) ....

Result ....

Test (specify) ....

Result ....

Test (specify) ....

Result ....

Test (specify) ....

Result ....

Test (specify) ....

Result ....

Immunizations, if any: ....

Treatments administered, if any: ....

Practitioner's observations/recommendations/answers to questions: ....

Your child's responses to recommended measures: ....

Other observations: ....

Questions to ask doctor at the next visit: ....

Child's name: .... Date of birth: ....

Well-baby visit number: .... Date: .... Baby's age: ....

Practitioner consulted: ....

General Physical Examination: ....

Weight: .... pounds .... ounces .... Length/height: .... inches .... Head circumference: .... inches

Other: ....

....

Developmental/behavioral evaluation: ....

Tests and screening procedures performed, if any: ....

    Test (specify) ....

    Result ....

    Test (specify) ....

    Result ....

    Test (specify) ....

    Result ....

    Test (specify) ....

    Result ....

    Test (specify) ....

    Result ....

Immunizations, if any: ....

....

Treatments administered, if any: ....

....

....

Practitioner's observations/recommendations/answers to questions: ....

....

....

Your child's responses to recommended measures: ....

....

....

Other observations: ....

....

Questions to ask doctor at the next visit: ....

....

Child's name: .... Date of birth: ....

Well-baby visit number: .... Date: .... Baby's age: ....

Practitioner consulted: ....

General Physical Examination: ....

Weight: .... pounds .... ounces .... Length/height: .... inches .... Head circumference: .... inches

Other: ....

Developmental/behavioral evaluation: ....

Tests and screening procedures performed, if any: ....

    Test (specify) ....

    Result ....

    Test (specify) ....

    Result ....

    Test (specify) ....

    Result ....

    Test (specify) ....

    Result ....

    Test (specify) ....

    Result ....

Immunizations, if any: ....

Treatments administered, if any: ....

....

Practitioner's observations/recommendations/answers to questions: ....

....

....

Your child's responses to recommended measures: ....

....

....

Other observations: ....

....

....

Questions to ask doctor at the next visit: ....

....

....

Child's name: .... Date of birth: ....

Well-baby visit number: .... Date: .... Baby's age: ....

Practitioner consulted: ....

General Physical Examination: ....

Weight: .... pounds .... ounces   Length/height: .... inches

Head circumference: .... inches   Other: ....

Developmental/behavioral evaluation: ....

Tests and screening procedures performed, if any: ....

     Test (specify) ....

     Result ....

     Test (specify) ....

     Result ....

     Test (specify) ....

     Result ....

     Test (specify) ....

     Result ....

     Test (specify) ....

     Result ....

Immunizations, if any: ....

Treatments administered, if any: ....

Practitioner's observations/recommendations/answers to questions: ....

Your child's responses to recommended measures: ....

Other observations: ....

Questions to ask doctor at the next visit: ....

The "Average" Baby?

At birth, most babies tip the scales at seven to eight pounds, and measure from nineteen to twenty-one inches long. But many factors influence these figures. If your baby weighs less or more, or is shorter or longer, it does not mean your child is less than perfect! There's no such thing as an "average" baby—each is a unique little person in his or her own right.

Child's name: .... Date of birth: ....

Well-baby visit number: .... Date: .... Baby's age: ....

Practitioner consulted: ....

General Physical Examination:

Weight: .... pounds .... ounces Length/height: .... inches Head circumference: .... inches

Other: ....
....

Developmental/behavioral evaluation: ....

Tests and screening procedures performed, if any:

    Test (specify) ....

    Result ....

    Test (specify) ....

    Result ....

    Test (specify) ....

    Result ....

    Test (specify) ....

    Result ....

    Test (specify) ....

    Result ....

Immunizations, if any: ....
....

Treatments administered, if any: ....
....
....

Practitioner's observations/recommendations/answers to questions: ....
....
....
....

Your child's responses to recommended measures: ....
....
....
....

Other observations: ....
....
....

Questions to ask doctor at the next visit: ....
....
....

Child's name: .... Date of birth: ....

Well-baby visit number: .... Date: .... Baby's age: ....

Practitioner consulted: ....

General Physical Examination: ....

Weight: .... pounds .... ounces Length/height: .... inches Head circumference: .... inches

Other: ....

....

Developmental/behavioral evaluation: ....

Tests and screening procedures performed, if any: ....

Test (specify) ....

Result ....

Test (specify) ....

Result ....

Test (specify) ....

Result ....

Test (specify) ....

Result ....

Test (specify) ....

Result ....

Immunizations, if any: ....

....

Treatments administered, if any: ....

....

....

Practitioner's observations/recommendations/answers to questions: ....

....

....

Your child's responses to recommended measures: ....

....

....

....

Other observations: ....

....

....

Questions to ask doctor at the next visit: ....

....

....

Ten Ways to Comfort a Crying Baby

If your baby is crying persistently, and there is no apparent reason, try to keep from becoming frantic. Stress and tension—both yours and your baby's—can make the problem worse. Instead, follow one or all of the following suggestions. Some babies respond to one; some (unfortunately) to none.

• Place your infant over your knees or against your chest with a warm-water bottle between you and your baby's stomach.

• If your baby loves water, try a warm, soothing splash in the bath.

• Massage your baby's stomach with a non-alcohol-based lotion or oil with a few drops of lavender oil added. Following the natural path of the intestines, gently rub from the lower right "corner" of the abdomen up across the bottom of the rib cage, down to the lower left "corner," and around again.

• Cuddle and/or rock your baby.

• Experiment to see whether being closely swaddled in a blanket or being under loose coverings that permit free movement suits your baby best.

Child's name:

Date of birth:

Well-baby visit number: Date: Baby's age:

Practitioner consulted:

General Physical Examination:

Weight: pounds   ounces   Length/height: inches

Head circumference: inches   Other:

Developmental/behavioral evaluation:

Tests and screening procedures performed, if any:

Test (specify)

Result

Test (specify)

Result

Test (specify)

Result

Test (specify)

Result

Test (specify)

Result

Immunizations, if any:

Treatments administered, if any:

Practitioner's observations/recommendations/answers to questions:

Your child's responses to recommended measures:

Other observations:

Questions to ask doctor at the next visit:

Child's name: ....

Date of birth: ....

Well-baby visit number: .... Date: .... Baby's age: ....

Practitioner consulted: ....

General Physical Examination:

Weight: .... pounds .... ounces Length/height: .... inches

Head circumference: .... inches Other: ....

Developmental/behavioral evaluation: ....

Tests and screening procedures performed, if any:

    Test (specify) ....

    Result ....

    Test (specify) ....

    Result ....

    Test (specify) ....

    Result ....

    Test (specify) ....

    Result ....

    Test (specify) ....

    Result ....

Immunizations, if any: ....

Treatments administered, if any: ....

Practitioner's observations/recommendations/answers to questions: ....

Your child's responses to recommended measures: ....

Other observations: ....

Questions to ask doctor at the next visit: ....

- Provide soft lighting, less touching, and a quiet atmosphere.

- Experiment with soft, comforting music; recordings of a heartbeat; and/or recordings of the sounds your baby lived with for nine months in the womb (interestingly, the sound of a washing machine often seems to have the same effect).

- Try vigorous movement. Putting on some lively music and bebopping around with babe in arms may not be your favorite 3:00 A.M. activity, but it's been known to work.

- Do "the bicycle" with your baby. With your baby lying on his or her back on the floor, gently move his or her legs in a bicycle-pedaling motion. Practice this exercise several times daily.

- Learn infant massage and practice it when your baby becomes fussy.

Finally, if your baby is prone to frequent crying spells and you feel your frustration is getting out of hand, talk to your health-care practitioner and seek emotional support and counseling for yourself.

Child's name: .... Date of birth: ....

Well-baby visit number: .... Date: .... Baby's age: ....

Practitioner consulted: ....

General Physical Examination: ....

Weight: .... pounds .... ounces Length/height: .... inches Head circumference: .... inches

Other: ....

....

Developmental/behavioral evaluation: ....

Tests and screening procedures performed, if any: ....

      Test (specify) ....

      Result ....

      Test (specify) ....

      Result ....

      Test (specify) ....

      Result ....

      Test (specify) ....

      Result ....

      Test (specify) ....

      Result ....

Immunizations, if any: ....

....

Treatments administered, if any: ....

....

....

Practitioner's observations/recommendations/answers to questions: ....

....

....

....

Your child's responses to recommended measures: ....

....

....

....

Other observations: ....

....

....

Questions to ask doctor at the next visit: ....

....

....

Child's name: .... Date of birth: ....

Well-baby visit number: .... Date: .... Baby's age: ....

Practitioner consulted: ....

General Physical Examination: ....

Weight: .... pounds .... ounces .... Length/height: .... inches .... Head circumference: .... inches

Other: ....
....

Developmental/behavioral evaluation: ....

Tests and screening procedures performed, if any: ....

     Test (specify) ....

     Result ....

     Test (specify) ....

     Result ....

     Test (specify) ....

     Result ....

     Test (specify) ....

     Result ....

     Test (specify) ....

     Result ....

Immunizations, if any: ....
....

Treatments administered, if any: ....
....
....

Practitioner's observations/recommendations/answers to questions: ....
....
....
....

Your child's responses to recommended measures: ....
....
....
....

Other observations: ....
....
....

Questions to ask doctor at the next visit: ....
....
....

Child's name: .... Date of birth: ....

Well-baby visit number: .... Date: .... Baby's age: ....

Practitioner consulted: ....

General Physical Examination:

Weight: .... pounds .... ounces Length/height: .... inches Head circumference: .... inches

Other: ....

Developmental/behavioral evaluation: ....

Tests and screening procedures performed, if any:

    Test (specify) ....

    Result ....

    Test (specify) ....

    Result ....

    Test (specify) ....

    Result ....

    Test (specify) ....

    Result ....

    Test (specify) ....

    Result ....

Immunizations, if any: ....

Treatments administered, if any: ....

....

Practitioner's observations/recommendations/answers to questions: ....

....

....

Your child's responses to recommended measures: ....

....

....

Other observations: ....

....

Questions to ask doctor at the next visit: ....

....

....

Child's name: .... Date of birth: ....

Well-baby visit number: .... Date: .... Baby's age: ....

Practitioner consulted: ....

General Physical Examination: ....

Weight: .... pounds .... ounces .... Length/height: .... inches .... Head circumference: .... inches

Other: ....

....

Developmental/behavioral evaluation: ....

Tests and screening procedures performed, if any: ....

    Test (specify) ....

    Result ....

    Test (specify) ....

    Result ....

    Test (specify) ....

    Result ....

    Test (specify) ....

    Result ....

    Test (specify) ....

    Result ....

Immunizations, if any: ....

....

Treatments administered, if any: ....

....

....

Practitioner's observations/recommendations/answers to questions: ....

....

....

....

Your child's responses to recommended measures: ....

....

....

Other observations: ....

....

....

Questions to ask doctor at the next visit: ....

....

....

PART THREE

FAMILY HEALTH RECORDS

Name: .... Date: ....

Symptoms and questions (be as specific as possible): ....

....

....

....

HEALTH-CARE VISIT

Practitioner consulted: ....

Tests and screening procedures performed, if any:

    Test (specify) ....

    Result ....

    Test (specify) ....

    Result ....

    Test (specify) ....

    Result ....

Treatments administered during the visit, if any: ....

....

Practitioner's observations/recommendations/answers to questions: ....

....

....

TREATMENTS USED

Conventional medicine:	Responses and observations:
Herbal medicine:	Responses and observations:
Homeopathic medicine:	Responses and observations:
Diet/nutritional supplements:	Responses and observations:
Other treatments/measures:	Responses and observations:

Follow-up Questions and Observations ....

....

....

....

Name: .... Date: ....

Symptoms and questions (be as specific as possible): ....

....

....

HEALTH-CARE VISIT

Practitioner consulted: ....

Tests and screening procedures performed, if any:

    Test (specify) ....

    Result ....

    Test (specify) ....

    Result ....

    Test (specify) ....

    Result ....

Treatments administered during the visit, if any: ....

Practitioner's observations/recommendations/answers to questions: ....

....

TREATMENTS USED

Conventional medicine: .... Responses and observations: ....

Herbal medicine: .... Responses and observations: ....

Homeopathic medicine: .... Responses and observations: ....

Diet/nutritional supplements: .... Responses and observations: ....

Other treatments/measures: .... Responses and observations: ....

Follow-up Questions and Observations ....

....

RECOMMENDED MEDICAL SCREENING TESTS FOR HEALTHY ADULTS

In addition to regular physical examinations, doctors recommend certain screening tests to check for problems that may not (or may not yet) be obvious in any other way. The table below summarizes some of the most commonly recommended tests and the usual frequency with which they are performed. Your doctor may order others as well, depending on your personal health history, your family history, or other factors, and may recommend more or less frequent testing than is indicated below, particularly if you have a chronic health problem.

Test	Performed
FOR MEN AND WOMEN	
Blood pressure	Age 18–35: Every 1–2 years. Age 36+: At every visit, at least every year.
Blood cholesterol and triglycerides	Age 18–35: Every 5 years. Age 36–50: Every 3 years. Age 50+: Every 2 years.
Complete blood count (including tests to measure thyroid, liver, and kidney function)	Age 18–35: Every 5 years. Age 36–50: Every 3 years. Age 50+: Every 2 years.
Fasting blood sugar	Age 18–35: Every 5 years (3 if high risk). Age 36–50: Every 3 years. Age 50+: Every 2 years.
Stool occult blood	Age 18–35: Every 5 years. Age 36–50: Every 3 years. Age 50+: Every year.
Digital rectal examination	Age 35+: Every year.
Sigmoidoscopy	Age 50+: Every 3–5 years.
FOR MEN ONLY	
Blood test for prostate-specific antigen	Age 50+: Every year.
FOR WOMEN ONLY	
Breast examination	Age 18–40: Every 3 years. Age 40+: Every year.
Mammogram	Age 35–40: Once (baseline). Age 40–49: Every 1–2 years. Age 50+: Every year.
Pelvic examination	Age 18–40: Every 1–3 years. Age 40+: Every year.
Pap test	Age 18–65: Every year.

Name: .... Date: ....

Symptoms and questions (be as specific as possible):
....
....
....

Health Spotlight: Fat and Cholesterol

- Cholesterol is actually a necessary nutrient. It is an important building block for vitamin D and for hormones from the adrenal glands and reproductive organs. It becomes a problem only if there is too much of it in the body.

- More important than your total cholesterol are the relative amounts of HDL ("good") and LDL ("bad") cholesterol in your blood. Even if your total cholesterol level is in the low to normal range, if your HDL level is low and your LDL level is high, you face an increased risk of cardiovasular disease and stroke.

- A diet high in cholesterol and saturated fat increases cholesterol levels. In fact, saturated fats may actually have a worse effect on cholesterol levels than foods that contain cholesterol.

HEALTH-CARE VISIT

Practitioner consulted: ....

Tests and screening procedures performed, if any:

Test (specify) ....

Result ....

Test (specify) ....

Result ....

Test (specify) ....

Result ....

Treatments administered during the visit, if any:
....

Practitioner's observations/recommendations/answers to questions:
....
....

TREATMENTS USED

Conventional medicine: .... Responses and observations: ....

Herbal medicine: .... Responses and observations: ....

Homeopathic medicine: .... Responses and observations: ....

Diet/nutritional supplements: .... Responses and observations: ....

Other treatments/measures: .... Responses and observations: ....

Follow-up Questions and Observations
....
....
....

Name: ....   Date: ....

Symptoms and questions (be as specific as possible):
....

....

....

HEALTH-CARE VISIT

Practitioner consulted: ....

Tests and screening procedures performed, if any:

    Test (specify) ....

    Result ....

    Test (specify) ....

    Result ....

    Test (specify) ....

    Result ....

Treatments administered during the visit, if any:
....

Practitioner's observations/recommendations/answers to questions:
....

....

- Trans-fatty acids, which are present in hydrogenated and partially hydrogenated oils (found in margarine, vegetable shortening, and many processed foods), have an effect on blood cholesterol that is similar to that of saturated fats.

- A diet high in fiber can reduce blood cholesterol. Eating garlic and onions regularly also can help to lower cholesterol.

- Regular exercise can improve your cholesterol profile, raising HDL and reducing LDL.

TREATMENTS USED

Conventional medicine: ....   Responses and observations: ....

....

....

Herbal medicine: ....   Responses and observations: ....

....

....

Homeopathic medicine: ....   Responses and observations: ....

....

....

Diet/nutritional supplements: ....   Responses and observations: ....

....

....

Other treatments/measures: ....   Responses and observations: ....

....

....

Follow-up Questions and Observations ....

....

....

....

Name: .... Date: ....

Symptoms and questions (be as specific as possible): ....

....

....

HEALTH-CARE VISIT

Practitioner consulted: ....

Tests and screening procedures performed, if any: ....

    Test (specify) ....

    Result ....

    Test (specify) ....

    Result ....

    Test (specify) ....

    Result ....

Treatments administered during the visit, if any: ....

....

Practitioner's observations/recommendations/answers to questions: ....

....

TREATMENTS USED

Conventional medicine: .... Responses and observations: ....

....

Herbal medicine: .... Responses and observations: ....

....

Homeopathic medicine: .... Responses and observations: ....

....

Diet/nutritional supplements: .... Responses and observations: ....

....

Other treatments/measures: .... Responses and observations: ....

....

Follow-up Questions and Observations

....

....

....

Name: .... Date: ....

Symptoms and questions (be as specific as possible): ....

....

....

HEALTH-CARE VISIT

Practitioner consulted: ....

Tests and screening procedures performed, if any:

    Test (specify) ....

    Result ....

    Test (specify) ....

    Result ....

    Test (specify) ....

    Result ....

Treatments administered during the visit, if any: ....

....

Practitioner's observations/recommendations/answers to questions: ....

....

....

TREATMENTS USED

Conventional medicine: ....   Responses and observations: ....

....

Herbal medicine: ....   Responses and observations: ....

....

Homeopathic medicine: ....   Responses and observations: ....

....

Diet/nutritional supplements: ....   Responses and observations: ....

....

Other treatments/measures: ....   Responses and observations: ....

....

Follow-up Questions and Observations ....

....

....

Name: .... Date: ....

Symptoms and questions (be as specific as possible): ....
....
....

Health Spotlight: Autoimmune Disease

Autoimmune diseases are disorders that come about because the immune system mistakenly begins to attack the body's own tissues. Why this happens is not well understood. Nor is it known why some people develop autoimmune disorders and others do not. The precise manifestation of autoimmune diseases may vary, depending on which type or types of tissues are damaged. Examples of disorders in which an autoimmune component is known or suspected include the following:

- Addison's disease
- Ankylosing spondylitis
- Glomerulonephritis
- Graves' disease
- Insulin resistance
- Multiple sclerosis
- Myasthenia gravis
- Pernicious anemia
- Rheumatoid arthritis
- Scleroderma
- Sjögren's syndrome
- Systemic lupus erythematosus
- Type 1 diabetes mellitus
- Some cases of infertility

Practitioner consulted: ....

Tests and screening procedures performed, if any:

    Test (specify) ....

    Result ....

    Test (specify) ....

    Result ....

    Test (specify) ....

    Result ....

Treatments administered during the visit, if any: ....
....

Practitioner's observations/recommendations/answers to questions: ....
....
....

TREATMENTS USED

Conventional medicine:	Responses and observations:
Herbal medicine:	Responses and observations:
Homeopathic medicine:	Responses and observations:
Diet/nutritional supplements:	Responses and observations:
Other treatments/measures:	Responses and observations:

Follow-up Questions and Observations
....
....
....

Name: .... Date: ....

Symptoms and questions (be as specific as possible): ....

....

....

HEALTH-CARE VISIT

Practitioner consulted: ....

Tests and screening procedures performed, if any:

    Test (specify) ....

    Result ....

    Test (specify) ....

    Result ....

    Test (specify) ....

    Result ....

Treatments administered during the visit, if any: ....

....

Practitioner's observations/recommendations/answers to questions: ....

....

....

TREATMENTS USED

Conventional medicine: .... Responses and observations: ....

....

Herbal medicine: .... Responses and observations: ....

....

Homeopathic medicine: .... Responses and observations: ....

....

Diet/nutritional supplements: .... Responses and observations: ....

....

Other treatments/measures: .... Responses and observations: ....

....

Follow-up Questions and Observations ....

....

....

Name: ....   Date: ....

Symptoms and questions (be as specific as possible): ....

....

....

HEALTH-CARE VISIT

Practitioner consulted: ....

Tests and screening procedures performed, if any: ....

    Test (specify) ....

    Result ....

    Test (specify) ....

    Result ....

    Test (specify) ....

    Result ....

Treatments administered during the visit, if any: ....

....

Practitioner's observations/recommendations/answers to questions: ....

....

....

TREATMENTS USED

Conventional medicine: ....   Responses and observations: ....

....

Herbal medicine: ....   Responses and observations: ....

....

Homeopathic medicine: ....   Responses and observations: ....

....

Diet/nutritional supplements: ....   Responses and observations: ....

....

Other treatments/measures: ....   Responses and observations: ....

....

....

Follow-up Questions and Observations ....

....

....

Name: .... Date: ....

Symptoms and questions (be as specific as possible): ....

....

....

HEALTH-CARE VISIT

Practitioner consulted: ....

Tests and screening procedures performed, if any:

    Test (specify) ....

    Result ....

    Test (specify) ....

    Result ....

    Test (specify) ....

    Result ....

Treatments administered during the visit, if any: ....

....

Practitioner's observations/recommendations/answers to questions: ....

....

TREATMENTS USED

Conventional medicine: .... Responses and observations: ....

Herbal medicine: .... Responses and observations: ....

Homeopathic medicine: .... Responses and observations: ....

Diet/nutritional supplements: .... Responses and observations: ....

Other treatments/measures: .... Responses and observations: ....

Follow-up Questions and Observations ....

....

"Prize" Vegetables

There are a number of vegetables that really stand out for the health-promoting nutrition they offer. Kale is one of them. A single 3.5-ounce serving of kale supplies nearly twice the recommended daily allowance of both vitamin A and vitamin C; 50 percent of the RDA of vitamin E; 15 to 20 percent of the RDA of vitamin B_6, folic acid, calcium, and iron; and 10 percent of the RDA of magnesium. Other "prize" vegetables include all of the members of the cabbage family, including red and green cabbage, savoy cabbage, bok choy, napa cabbage, broccoli, radishes, cauliflower, and Brussels sprouts.

Name: .... Date: ....

Symptoms and questions (be as specific as possible): ....

....

HEALTH-CARE VISIT

Practitioner consulted: ....

Tests and screening procedures performed, if any:

Test (specify) ....

Result ....

Test (specify) ....

Result ....

Test (specify) ....

Result ....

Treatments administered during the visit, if any: ....

....

Practitioner's observations/recommendations/answers to questions: ....

....

Health Spotlight: Humor and Healing

Laughter really is good medicine. Consider the following:

- It reduces levels of stress hormones in the body.

- It lessens depression and improves mood.

- It stimulates an increase in the activity of defensive immune cells, including T cells, that attack and kill tumor cells and viruses.

- It boosts the activity of antibodies that defend the body against harmful organisms.

- It steps up the production of interferon, a hormone that fights viruses and regulates cell growth.

TREATMENTS USED

Conventional medicine: .... Responses and observations: ....

....

Herbal medicine: .... Responses and observations: ....

....

Homeopathic medicine: .... Responses and observations: ....

....

Diet/nutritional supplements: .... Responses and observations: ....

....

Other treatments/measures: .... Responses and observations: ....

....

Follow-up Questions and Observations ....

....

....

Name: .... Date: ....

Symptoms and questions (be as specific as possible): ....

....

....

HEALTH-CARE VISIT

Practitioner consulted: ....

Tests and screening procedures performed, if any: ....

    Test (specify) ....

    Result ....

    Test (specify) ....

    Result ....

    Test (specify) ....

    Result ....

Treatments administered during the visit, if any: ....

....

Practitioner's observations/recommendations/answers to questions: ....

....

....

TREATMENTS USED

Conventional medicine: .... Responses and observations: ....

....

Herbal medicine: .... Responses and observations: ....

....

Homeopathic medicine: .... Responses and observations: ....

....

Diet/nutritional supplements: .... Responses and observations: ....

....

Other treatments/measures: .... Responses and observations: ....

....

Follow-up Questions and Observations ....

....

....

Name: .... Date: ....

Symptoms and questions (be as specific as possible): ....

....

....

HEALTH-CARE VISIT

Practitioner consulted: ....

Tests and screening procedures performed, if any:

      Test (specify) ....

      Result ....

      Test (specify) ....

      Result ....

      Test (specify) ....

      Result ....

Treatments administered during the visit, if any: ....

....

Practitioner's observations/recommendations/answers to questions: ....

....

....

TREATMENTS USED

Conventional medicine: ....   Responses and observations: ....

....

Herbal medicine: ....   Responses and observations: ....

....

Homeopathic medicine: ....   Responses and observations: ....

....

Diet/nutritional supplements: ....   Responses and observations: ....

....

Other treatments/measures: ....   Responses and observations: ....

....

....

Follow-up Questions and Observations ....

....

....

....

Name: .... Date: ....

Symptoms and questions (be as specific as possible):
....

....

....

HEALTH-CARE VISIT

Practitioner consulted: ....

Tests and screening procedures performed, if any:

    Test (specify) ....

    Result ....

    Test (specify) ....

    Result ....

    Test (specify) ....

    Result ....

Treatments administered during the visit, if any:
....

....

Practitioner's observations/recommendations/answers to questions:
....

....

TREATMENTS USED

Conventional medicine: ....   Responses and observations: ....

....

Herbal medicine: ....   Responses and observations: ....

....

Homeopathic medicine: ....   Responses and observations: ....

....

Diet/nutritional supplements: ....   Responses and observations: ....

....

Other treatments/measures: ....   Responses and observations: ....

....

Follow-up Questions and Observations
....

....

....

Health Spotlight: Back Pain

- More than 80 percent of Americans suffer from back pain at some point in their lives.

- Lower back pain (sometimes called *lumbago*) is the most common type of back pain.

- Back pain most often first strikes people in their thirties and may then recur, off and on, for the rest of their lives.

- Although advancing age and certain age-related health problems can cause backaches, back pain is not an inevitable part of aging.

- Most people blame their back pain on some kind of physical activity— twisting awkwardly or lifting something—but just as often, it comes on without any identifiable physical trigger.

- Most cases of back pain are caused by stress, muscle spasms, and/or muscular weakness, not problems with the spine.

Name: .... Date: ....

Symptoms and questions (be as specific as possible): ....

....

....

HEALTH-CARE VISIT

Health Spotlight: ADD/ADHD

- Although many parents of energetic children ask their doctors about attention deficit disorder/attention deficit hyperactivity disorder (ADD/ADHD), these are *not* common disorders. According to an article in the *British Journal of Psychiatry,* only 3 percent of children are actually diagnosed with ADD/ADHD.

- ADHD is ten times more common in boys than in girls.

- The exact cause or causes of ADD/ADHD are unknown. The medical community theorizes that these disorders may result from genetic factors; chemical imbalance; injury or disease at or after birth; or a defect in the brain or central nervous system, with the result that the mechanism responsible for controlling attention capabilities and filtering out extraneous stimuli does not work properly.

- As many as half of all children with ADD/ADHD have fewer behavior problems when put on a diet free of such substances as artificial flavorings, food colorings, preservatives, monosodium glutamate, caffeine, sugar, and chocolate.

Practitioner consulted: ....

Tests and screening procedures performed, if any:

    Test (specify) ....

    Result ....

    Test (specify) ....

    Result ....

    Test (specify) ....

    Result ....

Treatments administered during the visit, if any: ....

....

Practitioner's observations/recommendations/answers to questions: ....

....

TREATMENTS USED

Conventional medicine:	Responses and observations:
Herbal medicine:	Responses and observations:
Homeopathic medicine:	Responses and observations:
Diet/nutritional supplements:	Responses and observations:
Other treatments/measures:	Responses and observations:

Follow-up Questions and Observations ....

....

....

Name: .... Date: ....

Symptoms and questions (be as specific as possible):
....
....
....

HEALTH-CARE VISIT

Practitioner consulted: ....

Tests and screening procedures performed, if any:

    Test (specify) ....

    Result ....

    Test (specify) ....

    Result ....

    Test (specify) ....

    Result ....

Treatments administered during the visit, if any:
....
....

Practitioner's observations/recommendations/answers to questions:
....
....

TREATMENTS USED

Conventional medicine: Responses and observations:
....
....

Herbal medicine: Responses and observations:
....
....

Homeopathic medicine: Responses and observations:
....
....

Diet/nutritional supplements: Responses and observations:
....
....

Other treatments/measures: Responses and observations:
....
....
....

Follow-up Questions and Observations
....
....

Health Spotlight: Rescue Remedy

Rescue Remedy is probably the most popular of the Bach Flower Remedies. It is a premixed combination remedy made from the essences of cherry plum, clematis, impatiens, rock rose, and star of Bethlehem. It is useful in many crisis situations, such as after hearing bad news, before a major or anxiety-provoking event, or after an injury or nightmare. It helps to restore balance and relieve apprehension when you are nervous, panicked, or tense. Rescue Remedy is particularly good in acute situations when the cause of the distress is not clear—when you feel overwhelmed and/or intensely frustrated yet cannot say precisely why. When you are feeling stressed, put two or three drops of this remedy in half a glass of water and sip it slowly. Or just place a few drops under your tongue.

Name: .... Date: ....

Symptoms and questions (be as specific as possible): ....

....

....

HEALTH-CARE VISIT

Practitioner consulted: ....

Tests and screening procedures performed, if any:

Test (specify) ....

Result ....

Test (specify) ....

Result ....

Test (specify) ....

Result ....

Treatments administered during the visit, if any: ....

Practitioner's observations/recommendations/answers to questions: ....

....

....

TREATMENTS USED

Conventional medicine: .... Responses and observations: ....

Herbal medicine: .... Responses and observations: ....

Homeopathic medicine: .... Responses and observations: ....

Diet/nutritional supplements: .... Responses and observations: ....

Other treatments/measures: .... Responses and observations: ....

Follow-up Questions and Observations ....

....

....

Name: .... Date: ....

Symptoms and questions (be as specific as possible): ....

....

....

HEALTH-CARE VISIT

Practitioner consulted: ....

Tests and screening procedures performed, if any:

    Test (specify) ....

    Result ....

    Test (specify) ....

    Result ....

    Test (specify) ....

    Result ....

Treatments administered during the visit, if any: ....

....

Practitioner's observations/recommendations/answers to questions: ....

....

....

TREATMENTS USED

Conventional medicine: .... | Responses and observations: ....

Herbal medicine: .... | Responses and observations: ....

Homeopathic medicine: .... | Responses and observations: ....

Diet/nutritional supplements: .... | Responses and observations: ....

Other treatments/measures: .... | Responses and observations: ....

Follow-up Questions and Observations ....

....

....

Health Spotlight: Breast Cancer

- Breast cancer is the most common type of cancer in women.

- Breast cancer can occur at any age (after puberty), but is most often found in women over the age of fifty.

- The majority of breast cancers occur in the upper outer quadrant of the breast.

- 70 to 80 percent of all breast cancers are infiltrating (or invasive) ductal carcinomas, 6 to 8 percent are invasive lobular carcinomas, and 4 to 6 percent are noninvasive lobular and intraductal carcinomas.

- The precise cause or causes of breast cancer are not well understood, but factors associated with a higher than average risk of the disease include a family history of breast cancer, early menarche (onset of menstrual cycles), late menopause, late childbearing, and obesity. About 5 percent of breast cancer cases are thought to be related to an abnormality in a single gene, BRCA1. However, more than 70 percent of women who develop breast cancer have no known risk factors.

- Men also can get breast cancer.

- When detected early, most breast cancers are considered 70 to 90 percent curable.

Name: .... Date: ....

Symptoms and questions (be as specific as possible): ....
....
....
....

HEALTH-CARE VISIT

Health Spotlight: Are You Getting Enough Sleep?

At the beginning of the twentieth century, Americans slept an average of nine hours a night. That figure has now dropped to seven hours a night. This is fine for some people, but insufficient for many. To assess your personal sleep needs, consider the following:

- How long does it take you to fall asleep? If you drop off within five minutes, you may not be getting enough sleep.

- Do you sleep through the night or toss restlessly and wake up repeatedly? If the latter, you may not be getting the quality sleep you need.

Practitioner consulted: ....

Tests and screening procedures performed, if any:

Test (specify) ....

Result ....

Test (specify) ....

Result ....

Test (specify) ....

Result ....

Treatments administered during the visit, if any: ....
....

Practitioner's observations/recommendations/answers to questions: ....
....
....

TREATMENTS USED

Conventional medicine: ....   Responses and observations: ....
....

Herbal medicine: ....   Responses and observations: ....
....

Homeopathic medicine: ....   Responses and observations: ....
....

Diet/nutritional supplements: ....   Responses and observations: ....
....

Other treatments/measures: ....   Responses and observations: ....
....
....

Follow-up Questions and Observations
....
....

Name: .... Date: ....

Symptoms and questions (be as specific as possible):
....
....
....

HEALTH-CARE VISIT

Practitioner consulted: ....

Tests and screening procedures performed, if any:

    Test (specify) ....

    Result ....

    Test (specify) ....

    Result ....

    Test (specify) ....

    Result ....

Treatments administered during the visit, if any:
....

Practitioner's observations/recommendations/answers to questions:
....
....

TREATMENTS USED

Conventional medicine: Responses and observations:

Herbal medicine: Responses and observations:

Homeopathic medicine: Responses and observations:

Diet/nutritional supplements: Responses and observations:

Other treatments/measures: Responses and observations:

Follow-up Questions and Observations
....
....

- Does the alarm clock jar you out of a sound sleep? If so, chances are you are building up a sleep deficit. If you have had enough sleep, you will awaken naturally.

- How rested do you feel upon awakening? Are you alert and active during the waking hours? If you have slept long enough to truly restore your body, you should find it almost impossible to nap during the daylight hours.

Lack of sleep fogs the memory, reduces alertness, lengthens reaction time, dims the creative spark, and can even twist your tongue. On top of all that, when you force your body to function without enough sleep, your ability to resist illness and disease declines. No matter how wholesome your diet and regular your exercise routine, you cannot be truly healthy and at your best without sufficient, regular good-quality sleep.

Name: .... Date: ....

Symptoms and questions (be as specific as possible): ....

....

....

HEALTH-CARE VISIT

Practitioner consulted: ....

Tests and screening procedures performed, if any:

    Test (specify) ....

    Result ....

    Test (specify) ....

    Result ....

    Test (specify) ....

    Result ....

Treatments administered during the visit, if any: ....

....

Practitioner's observations/recommendations/answers to questions: ....

....

....

TREATMENTS USED

Conventional medicine: .... Responses and observations: ....

Herbal medicine: .... Responses and observations: ....

Homeopathic medicine: .... Responses and observations: ....

Diet/nutritional supplements: .... Responses and observations: ....

Other treatments/measures: .... Responses and observations: ....

Follow-up Questions and Observations ....

....

....

Name: .... Date: ....

Symptoms and questions (be as specific as possible): ....

....

....

HEALTH-CARE VISIT

Practitioner consulted: ....

Tests and screening procedures performed, if any: ....

    Test (specify) ....

    Result ....

    Test (specify) ....

    Result ....

    Test (specify) ....

    Result ....

Treatments administered during the visit, if any: ....

....

Practitioner's observations/recommendations/answers to questions: ....

....

....

TREATMENTS USED

Conventional medicine: .... Responses and observations: ....

....

Herbal medicine: .... Responses and observations: ....

....

Homeopathic medicine: .... Responses and observations: ....

....

Diet/nutritional supplements: .... Responses and observations: ....

....

Other treatments/measures: .... Responses and observations: ....

....

Follow-up Questions and Observations ....

....

....

Name: .... Date: ....

Symptoms and questions (be as specific as possible):
....

....

....

HEALTH-CARE VISIT

Health Spotlight: Food Cravings

Practitioner consulted: ....

Tests and screening procedures performed, if any:

- Cravings for sweets often relect blood-sugar imbalances and a desire for a "quick-fix" stimulant. The mineral chromium, the herbs astragalus and *Garcinia cambogia,* and homeopathic *Lycopodium* can help.

    Test (specify) ....

    Result ....

    Test (specify) ....

    Result ....

    Test (specify) ....

    Result ....

Treatments administered during the visit, if any:
....

- Cravings for fatty foods are often a sign that you are eating the wrong kinds of fats and/or not digesting fat properly. Try taking supplemental flaxseed oil or the herb *Garcinia cambogia.*

Practitioner's observations/recommendations/answers to questions:
....

....

- Cravings for chocolate may be due to the fact that it is a mild stimulant and mood elevator (and it tastes good), but also may be related to a deficiency of chromium and/or magnesium. When these nutrients are provided, cravings often become manageable. A Chinese herbal formula called bu zhong yi qu wan also can diminish chocolate cravings.

TREATMENTS USED

Conventional medicine: Responses and observations:

Herbal medicine: Responses and observations:

Homeopathic medicine: Responses and observations:

Diet/nutritional supplements: Responses and observations:

Other treatments/measures: Responses and observations:

Follow-up Questions and Observations
....

....

....

Name: _____   Date: _____

Symptoms and questions (be as specific as possible):
....
....
....

HEALTH-CARE VISIT

Practitioner consulted: ....

Tests and screening procedures performed, if any:

    Test (specify) ....

    Result ....

    Test (specify) ....

    Result ....

    Test (specify) ....

    Result ....

Treatments administered during the visit, if any:
....
....

Practitioner's observations/recommendations/answers to questions:
....
....

TREATMENTS USED

Conventional medicine:	Responses and observations:

Herbal medicine:	Responses and observations:

Homeopathic medicine:	Responses and observations:

Diet/nutritional supplements:	Responses and observations:

Other treatments/measures:	Responses and observations:

Follow-up Questions and Observations
....
....
....

- Cravings for salty foods are most often not a sign of nutritional deficiency, but of taste buds that have been accustomed to the overuse of salt from childhood on. You can retrain your taste buds by slowly cutting back on your consumption of salt over a period of weeks. Or try using kelp powder instead of salt. Kelp is a naturally salty-tasting sea vegetable that is nevertheless low in sodium.

- If you're always hungry, you are probably not eating the right kinds of foods. Increase your intake of high-fiber foods; eat small, more frequent meals; and try supplemental chromium and/or the herb *Garcinia cambogia*.

Name: .... Date: ....

Symptoms and questions (be as specific as possible): ....
....
....
....

HEALTH-CARE VISIT

Practitioner consulted: ....

Tests and screening procedures performed, if any:

    Test (specify) ....

    Result ....

    Test (specify) ....

    Result ....

    Test (specify) ....

    Result ....

Treatments administered during the visit, if any: ....
....

Practitioner's observations/recommendations/answers to questions: ....
....
....

TREATMENTS USED

Conventional medicine: .... Responses and observations: ....
....

Herbal medicine: .... Responses and observations: ....
....

Homeopathic medicine: .... Responses and observations: ....
....

Diet/nutritional supplements: .... Responses and observations: ....
....

Other treatments/measures: .... Responses and observations: ....
....
....

Follow-up Questions and Observations
....
....
....

Name: . . . . Date: . . . .

Symptoms and questions (be as specific as possible): . . . .

. . . .

. . . .

HEALTH-CARE VISIT

Practitioner consulted: . . . .

Tests and screening procedures performed, if any:

    Test (specify) . . . .

    Result . . . .

    Test (specify) . . . .

    Result . . . .

    Test (specify) . . . .

    Result . . . .

Treatments administered during the visit, if any: . . . .

. . . .

Practitioner's observations/recommendations/answers to questions: . . . .

. . . .

. . . .

TREATMENTS USED

Conventional medicine:	Responses and observations:
Herbal medicine:	Responses and observations:
Homeopathic medicine:	Responses and observations:
Diet/nutritional supplements:	Responses and observations:
Other treatments/measures:	Responses and observations:

Follow-up Questions and Observations . . . .

. . . .

. . . .

Name: .... Date: ....

Symptoms and questions (be as specific as possible): ....

....

....

Health Spotlight: Carpal Tunnel Syndrome

- Carpal tunnel syndrome (CTS) gets its name from the medical term for a narrow gap under a ligament at the front of the wrist, through which the median nerve carries messages between the thumb and some of the fingers to the brain.

- Most cases of CTS are due to repetitive stress injury (making certain types of repetitive motions of the wrist, which causes inflammation and pressure on the median nerve).

- Repetitive stress injuries currently account for more than 60 percent of the work-related illnesses reported in the United States.

- With the advent of the computer age, the number of repetitive stress injuries has been increasing by some 10 percent each year.

HEALTH-CARE VISIT

Practitioner consulted: ....

Tests and screening procedures performed, if any:

Test (specify) ....

Result ....

Test (specify) ....

Result ....

Test (specify) ....

Result ....

Treatments administered during the visit, if any: ....

....

Practitioner's observations/recommendations/answers to questions: ....

....

TREATMENTS USED

Conventional medicine: ....   Responses and observations: ....

....

Herbal medicine: ....   Responses and observations: ....

....

Homeopathic medicine: ....   Responses and observations: ....

....

Diet/nutritional supplements: ....   Responses and observations: ....

....

Other treatments/measures: ....   Responses and observations: ....

....

Follow-up Questions and Observations

....

....

....

Name: .... Date: ....

Symptoms and questions (be as specific as possible): ....

....

....

HEALTH-CARE VISIT

Practitioner consulted: ....

Tests and screening procedures performed, if any:

    Test (specify) ....

    Result ....

    Test (specify) ....

    Result ....

    Test (specify) ....

    Result ....

Treatments administered during the visit, if any: ....

....

Practitioner's observations/recommendations/answers to questions: ....

....

TREATMENTS USED

Conventional medicine:	Responses and observations:
Herbal medicine:	Responses and observations:
Homeopathic medicine:	Responses and observations:
Diet/nutritional supplements:	Responses and observations:
Other treatments/measures:	Responses and observations:

Follow-up Questions and Observations

....

....

....

- CTS occurs most often in middle-aged women. It occurs more often than usual in women who have just started taking birth control pills, pregnant women, and women who suffer from premenstrual syndrome. Arthritis sufferers of both sexes also seem more likely to be afflicted than other people.

- Data entry and cashiering are well-known causes of CTS, but it can also be caused by writing, small-parts assembly, guitar-playing, knitting, crocheting, and even playing tennis. Chefs who spend hours each day cutting and chopping sometimes suffer from carpal tunnel syndrome as well.

Name: .... Date: ....

Symptoms and questions (be as specific as possible):
....
....
....

HEALTH-CARE VISIT

Health Spotlight: The Pap Smear

- The Pap smear was named for George Papanicolaou, the physician who developed it.

- A woman should have a routine Pap smear at age eighteen or within six months of first having sexual intercourse, whichever comes first, and another within the following six to twelve months. Thereafter, ideally, a Pap smear should be a regular part of a yearly checkup.

- The Pap smear offers a 95-percent chance of detecting cervical dysplasia, which is the best means of preventing cervical cancer. Pap smears are also useful for identifying viral infections of the cervix, such as herpes simplex and papillomavirus infection.

Practitioner consulted: ....

Tests and screening procedures performed, if any:

Test (specify) ....

Result ....

Test (specify) ....

Result ....

Test (specify) ....

Result ....

Treatments administered during the visit, if any:
....
....

Practitioner's observations/recommendations/answers to questions:
....
....

TREATMENTS USED

Conventional medicine: .... Responses and observations: ....
....

Herbal medicine: .... Responses and observations: ....
....

Homeopathic medicine: .... Responses and observations: ....
....

Diet/nutritional supplements: .... Responses and observations: ....
....

Other treatments/measures: .... Responses and observations: ....
....
....

Follow-up Questions and Observations
....
....
....

Name: .... Date: ....

Symptoms and questions (be as specific as possible): ....

....

....

HEALTH-CARE VISIT

Practitioner consulted: ....

Tests and screening procedures performed, if any:

    Test (specify) ....

    Result ....

    Test (specify) ....

    Result ....

    Test (specify) ....

    Result ....

Treatments administered during the visit, if any: ....

....

Practitioner's observations/recommendations/answers to questions: ....

....

....

TREATMENTS USED

Conventional medicine:	Responses and observations:
Herbal medicine:	Responses and observations:
Homeopathic medicine:	Responses and observations:
Diet/nutritional supplements:	Responses and observations:
Other treatments/measures:	Responses and observations:

Follow-up Questions and Observations

....

....

....

Name: .... Date: ....

Symptoms and questions (be as specific as possible):
....
....
....

Health Spotlight: The Common Cold

- Average, otherwise healthy adults usually have no more than two colds a year. Because their immune systems are still developing, children under six years of age have an average of seven colds a year, and older children have four or five.

- Most colds occur during the winter months, from October through February.

- A cold is most contagious in its early phase, when nasal secretions are thin, watery mucus that is almost entirely composed of viral discharge. It becomes less contagious when the secretions turn thick and yellowish or greenish, evidence of the presence of dead white blood cells, dead viral particles, and dead bacteria.

- By themselves, most colds do not cause significant fever in otherwise healthy adults. In children, this is less predictable.

HEALTH-CARE VISIT

Practitioner consulted: ....

Tests and screening procedures performed, if any:

    Test (specify) ....

    Result ....

    Test (specify) ....

    Result ....

    Test (specify) ....

    Result ....

Treatments administered during the visit, if any:
....

Practitioner's observations/recommendations/answers to questions:
....
....

TREATMENTS USED

Conventional medicine:	Responses and observations:
Herbal medicine:	Responses and observations:
Homeopathic medicine:	Responses and observations:
Diet/nutritional supplements:	Responses and observations:
Other treatments/measures:	Responses and observations:

Follow-up Questions and Observations
....
....
....

Name: .... Date: ....

Symptoms and questions (be as specific as possible):
....

....

....

HEALTH-CARE VISIT

Practitioner consulted: ....

Tests and screening procedures performed, if any:

Test (specify) ....

Result ....

Test (specify) ....

Result ....

Test (specify) ....

Result ....

Treatments administered during the visit, if any:
....

....

Practitioner's observations/recommendations/answers to questions:
....

....

- Antibiotics are ineffective against viruses and therefore can do nothing to cure the common cold. In fact, they may hinder healing by destroying the healthy bacteria normally present in the respiratory tract, giving the cold virus more room to multiply.

- From start to finish, the average common cold, if uncomplicated, lasts about five to ten days. If you are sick for more than fourteen days in a row, you may have a different illness or have contracted a series of viruses.

TREATMENTS USED

Conventional medicine: Responses and observations:
....

....

Herbal medicine: Responses and observations:
....

....

Homeopathic medicine: Responses and observations:
....

....

Diet/nutritional supplements: Responses and observations:
....

....

Other treatments/measures: Responses and observations:
....

....

Follow-up Questions and Observations
....

....

....

Name: .... Date: ....

Symptoms and questions (be as specific as possible): ....

....

....

HEALTH-CARE VISIT

Practitioner consulted: ....

Tests and screening procedures performed, if any: ....

      Test (specify) ....

      Result ....

      Test (specify) ....

      Result ....

      Test (specify) ....

      Result ....

Treatments administered during the visit, if any: ....

....

Practitioner's observations/recommendations/answers to questions: ....

....

....

TREATMENTS USED

Conventional medicine:	Responses and observations: ....
....	....
Herbal medicine:	Responses and observations: ....
....	....
Homeopathic medicine:	Responses and observations: ....
....	....
Diet/nutritional supplements:	Responses and observations: ....
....	....
Other treatments/measures:	Responses and observations: ....
....	....
....	....

Follow-up Questions and Observations ....

....

....

Name: .... Date: ....

Symptoms and questions (be as specific as possible): ....

....

....

HEALTH-CARE VISIT

Practitioner consulted: ....

Tests and screening procedures performed, if any:

    Test (specify) ....

    Result ....

    Test (specify) ....

    Result ....

    Test (specify) ....

    Result ....

Treatments administered during the visit, if any: ....

....

Practitioner's observations/recommendations/answers to questions: ....

....

TREATMENTS USED

Conventional medicine:	Responses and observations:
Herbal medicine:	Responses and observations:
Homeopathic medicine:	Responses and observations:
Diet/nutritional supplements:	Responses and observations:
Other treatments/measures:	Responses and observations:

Follow-up Questions and Observations ....

....

....

Health Spotlight: Aromatherapy for Stress

Aromatherapy is one of the best, and most pleasurable, natural ways of reducing stress. This healing art utilizes essential oils, which are intensely concentrated extracts of plants, to stimulate beneficial changes within the body. It is important to use 100-percent pure essential oils, not merely fragrant oils. When you're feeling stressed out, treat yourself to a bath with 10 to 20 drops of essential oil added. Or merely inhale straight from the bottle. Some of the essential oils most renowned for stress reduction include the following:

- Bergamot (*Citrus bergamia*)

- Chamomile (*Chamaemelum nobile, Matricaria chamomilla,* or *Anthemis mixta*)

- Clary Sage (*Salvia sclarea*)

- Elemi (*Canarium luzonicum*)

- Lavender (*Lavandula officinalis*)

- Neroli (*Citrus aurantium, Citrus bigaradia,* or *Citrus vulgaris*)

- Rose (*Rosa damascena* or *Rosa gallica*)

- Ylang ylang (*Cananga odorata*)

HEALTH SPOTLIGHT:
DAILY FLUID REQUIREMENTS

Many people suffer from chronic, low-level dehydration simply because they fail to take in sufficient fluids. This can lead to chronic constipation, weight gain, elevated cholesterol levels, a decreased threshold of pain, and a decreased ability to clear toxins from the body. The table below gives an approximation of appropriate liquid intake by age.

Age	Recommended Fluid Intake
Infant	1½–5½ cups
School-age child	6–7½ cups
Adolescent	9–11½ cups
Adult (by body weight):	
100 lbs.	10–12 cups
125 lbs.	10½–12½ cups
150 lbs.	11–13 cups
175 lbs.	11½–13½ cups
200 lbs.	12–14 cups

Name: ....   Date: ....

Symptoms and questions (be as specific as possible): ....

....

....

HEALTH-CARE VISIT

Practitioner consulted: ....

Tests and screening procedures performed, if any:

    Test (specify) ....

    Result ....

    Test (specify) ....

    Result ....

    Test (specify) ....

    Result ....

Treatments administered during the visit, if any: ....

....

Practitioner's observations/recommendations/answers to questions: ....

....

....

TREATMENTS USED

Conventional medicine: ....   Responses and observations: ....

....

Herbal medicine: ....   Responses and observations: ....

....

Homeopathic medicine: ....   Responses and observations: ....

....

Diet/nutritional supplements: ....   Responses and observations: ....

....

Other treatments/measures: ....   Responses and observations: ....

....

Follow-up Questions and Observations ....

....

....

Name: .... Date: ....

Symptoms and questions (be as specific as possible):
....
....
....

HEALTH-CARE VISIT

Practitioner consulted: ....

Tests and screening procedures performed, if any:

Test (specify) ....

Result ....

Test (specify) ....

Result ....

Test (specify) ....

Result ....

Treatments administered during the visit, if any:
....
....

Practitioner's observations/recommendations/answers to questions:
....

Health Spotlight: Diabetes

The American Diabetes Association estimates that there are 8 million Americans who are unaware they have diabetes. Early diagnosis means that treatment can begin before the disease causes damage to the eyes, heart, kidneys, and nerves. To assess your personal risk of developing diabetes, take the following test and add up the results:

- *I weigh at least 20 percent more than is recommended for a medium-framed person of my height.*
  True = 5 points   False = 0 points

- *I am under age sixty-five, and I get little or no exercise during a usual day.*
  True = 5 points   False = 0 points

- *I am a woman who has had a baby weighing more than 9 pounds at birth.*
  True = 1 point   False = 0 points

- *I have a sister or brother with diabetes.*
  True = 1 point   False = 0 points

- *I have a parent with diabetes.*
  True = 1 point   False = 0 points

If your score adds up to between 3 and 9 points, your risk of diabetes is low. If your score is 10 or more, you are at high risk. Consult with your health-care provider.

TREATMENTS USED

Conventional medicine: .... Responses and observations: ....

Herbal medicine: .... Responses and observations: ....

Homeopathic medicine: .... Responses and observations: ....

Diet/nutritional supplements: .... Responses and observations: ....

Other treatments/measures: .... Responses and observations: ....

Follow-up Questions and Observations
....
....
....

Name: .... Date: ....

Symptoms and questions (be as specific as possible): ....

....

....

HEALTH-CARE VISIT

Practitioner consulted: ....

Tests and screening procedures performed, if any:

    Test (specify) ....

    Result ....

    Test (specify) ....

    Result ....

    Test (specify) ....

    Result ....

Treatments administered during the visit, if any: ....

....

Practitioner's observations/recommendations/answers to questions: ....

....

....

TREATMENTS USED

Conventional medicine:	Responses and observations:
Herbal medicine:	Responses and observations:
Homeopathic medicine:	Responses and observations:
Diet/nutritional supplements:	Responses and observations:
Other treatments/measures:	Responses and observations:

Follow-up Questions and Observations

....

....

....

Name: .... Date: ....

Symptoms and questions (be as specific as possible): ....

....

....

HEALTH-CARE VISIT

Practitioner consulted: ....

Tests and screening procedures performed, if any:

    Test (specify) ....

    Result ....

    Test (specify) ....

    Result ....

    Test (specify) ....

    Result ....

Treatments administered during the visit, if any: ....

....

Practitioner's observations/recommendations/answers to questions: ....

....

....

TREATMENTS USED

Conventional medicine: ....   Responses and observations: ....

....

Herbal medicine: ....   Responses and observations: ....

....

Homeopathic medicine: ....   Responses and observations: ....

....

Diet/nutritional supplements: ....   Responses and observations: ....

....

Other treatments/measures: ....   Responses and observations: ....

....

Follow-up Questions and Observations ....

....

....

HEALTH SPOTLIGHT:
WARNING SIGNS OF DRUG ABUSE

Different drugs have different effects on the body and mind. The table below outlines common signs of abuse that occur with different classes of drugs.

Type of Drug	Signs of Abuse
Amphetamines ("uppers" or "speed")	Abnormally high energy level, dilated pupils, weight loss, insomnia
Antianxiety drugs, tranquilizers, sleeping pills ("downers")	Lack of interest, slurred speech, poor balance, constricted pupils, excessive need for sleep
Cocaine, crack	Inhaled: Ulcerated nostrils Injected: Needle tracks Smoked: Runny nose, sniffles
Hallucinogens (lysergic acid diethylamide [LSD], mescaline [peyote], some "designer" drugs)	Unpredictable hallucinations, sometimes pleasant, sometimes frightening; dilated pupils; irregular heart rate
Inhalants (volatile fumes from glue or cleaning fluids)	Unpredictable hallucinations, euphoria, silliness, dilated pupils
Marijuana (pot), hashish (hash)	Red eyes, dilated pupils, excessive "goofiness," mood swings, abnormally slow reflexes and sense of time, increased appetite
Opiates (heroin, opium, morphine)	Mood swings, sweating, slurred speech, drowsiness, weight loss, lethargy

Name: .... Date: ....

Symptoms and questions (be as specific as possible): ....

....

....

HEALTH-CARE VISIT

Practitioner consulted: ....

Tests and screening procedures performed, if any:

    Test (specify) ....

    Result ....

    Test (specify) ....

    Result ....

    Test (specify) ....

    Result ....

Treatments administered during the visit, if any: ....

Practitioner's observations/recommendations/answers to questions: ....

....

....

TREATMENTS USED

Conventional medicine: ....   Responses and observations: ....

Herbal medicine: ....   Responses and observations: ....

Homeopathic medicine: ....   Responses and observations: ....

Diet/nutritional supplements: ....   Responses and observations: ....

Other treatments/measures: ....   Responses and observations: ....

Follow-up Questions and Observations ....

....

....

Name: .... Date: ....

Symptoms and questions (be as specific as possible): ....

....

....

HEALTH-CARE VISIT

Practitioner consulted: ....

Tests and screening procedures performed, if any:

    Test (specify) ....

    Result ....

    Test (specify) ....

    Result ....

    Test (specify) ....

    Result ....

Treatments administered during the visit, if any: ....

....

Practitioner's observations/recommendations/answers to questions: ....

....

TREATMENTS USED

Conventional medicine:	Responses and observations:
Herbal medicine:	Responses and observations:
Homeopathic medicine:	Responses and observations:
Diet/nutritional supplements:	Responses and observations:
Other treatments/measures:	Responses and observations:

Follow-up Questions and Observations ....

....

Health Spotlight: Childhood Ear Infections

- Every year, more than 10 million children in the United States are treated for middle ear infections.

- Ear infections are most common in young children between six months and three years of age. They are often a complication of an upper respiratory infection such as a cold or an infection of the adenoids, tonsils, or sinuses.

- Most children outgrow ear infections as their bodies mature and the shape of the structure of the middle ear changes.

- While antibiotics are a common treatment for ear infections, it is interesting to note that a study done in the Netherlands found that while children given antibiotics for ear infections improved somewhat faster than those given a placebo, there was little difference between the two groups in long-term outcome.

Name:

Date:

Symptoms and questions (be as specific as possible):

Health Spotlight: Hair Loss

- Individual hairs do not grow continuously. Rather, each hair goes through an anagen (or growth) phase, followed by a telogen (or resting) phase, after which it is shed and the process begins again.

- It is normal to lose up to fifty scalp hairs a day as the follicles go through their cycles. Hair loss occurs if enough follicles fail to produce new hairs after the old ones have been shed.

- The most common type of hair loss is male pattern baldness, which is linked both to heredity and to high testosterone levels. Interestingly, although it is predominantly a male problem, it appears to be passed on by the mother.

HEALTH-CARE VISIT

Practitioner consulted:

Tests and screening procedures performed, if any:

Test (specify)

Result

Test (specify)

Result

Test (specify)

Result

Treatments administered during the visit, if any:

Practitioner's observations/recommendations/answers to questions:

TREATMENTS USED

Conventional medicine:

Responses and observations:

Herbal medicine:

Responses and observations:

Homeopathic medicine:

Responses and observations:

Diet/nutritional supplements:

Responses and observations:

Other treatments/measures:

Responses and observations:

Follow-up Questions and Observations

Name: .... Date: ....

Symptoms and questions (be as specific as possible): ....

....

....

HEALTH-CARE VISIT

Practitioner consulted: ....

Tests and screening procedures performed, if any:

    Test (specify) ....

    Result ....

    Test (specify) ....

    Result ....

    Test (specify) ....

    Result ....

Treatments administered during the visit, if any: ....

....

Practitioner's observations/recommendations/answers to questions: ....

....

....

- Women also can develop hormone-related hair loss, usually at times when hormone levels are shifting significantly, such as after menopause and during and after pregnancy. Women generally experience this kind of hair loss primarily as a thinning of the hair, and hair loss is not as extensive as it is for men.

- Other causes of hair loss include infection, scarring or atrophy of the follicles, and certain drugs, especially cancer chemotherapy agents. Sometimes hair loss occurs for no identifiable reason.

TREATMENTS USED

Conventional medicine:	Responses and observations:

Herbal medicine:	Responses and observations:

Homeopathic medicine:	Responses and observations:

Diet/nutritional supplements:	Responses and observations:

Other treatments/measures:	Responses and observations:

Follow-up Questions and Observations

....

....

....

Name: .... Date: ....

Symptoms and questions (be as specific as possible): ....

....

....

HEALTH-CARE VISIT

Practitioner consulted: ....

Tests and screening procedures performed, if any:

    Test (specify) ....

    Result ....

    Test (specify) ....

    Result ....

    Test (specify) ....

    Result ....

Treatments administered during the visit, if any: ....

....

Practitioner's observations/recommendations/answers to questions: ....

....

....

TREATMENTS USED

Conventional medicine: ....   Responses and observations: ....

....

Herbal medicine: ....   Responses and observations: ....

....

Homeopathic medicine: ....   Responses and observations: ....

....

Diet/nutritional supplements: ....   Responses and observations: ....

....

Other treatments/measures: ....   Responses and observations: ....

....

Follow-up Questions and Observations ....

....

....

Name: .... Date: ....

Symptoms and questions (be as specific as possible): ....

....

....

HEALTH-CARE VISIT

Practitioner consulted: ....

Tests and screening procedures performed, if any: ....

    Test (specify) ....

    Result ....

    Test (specify) ....

    Result ....

    Test (specify) ....

    Result ....

Treatments administered during the visit, if any: ....

....

Practitioner's observations/recommendations/answers to questions: ....

....

TREATMENTS USED

Conventional medicine:	Responses and observations:
Herbal medicine:	Responses and observations:
Homeopathic medicine:	Responses and observations:
Diet/nutritional supplements:	Responses and observations:
Other treatments/measures:	Responses and observations:

Follow-up Questions and Observations

....

....

Health Spotlight: Herbal Treatment for Headaches

Aspirin, the classic conventional medication for headaches, was originally derived from white willow bark and the meadowsweet plant. There are a number of other herbal treatments that can be effective for headaches as well, including the following:

- Tincture of arnica, used as a rub and massaged into the temples and/or forehead. Be very careful to keep tinctures away from your eyes, and do not use them on broken skin.

- Chamomile and/or passionflower tea, either taken internally or used to prepare an herbal bath. These herbs can tame a tension headache.

- Feverfew, taken in the form of freeze-dried extract. Taken regularly, this herb can ward off migraines.

- Ginger and/or peppermint tea. These are helpful for a tension headache, a migraine concentrated in the front of the head, a congested and full headache, and/or a headache caused by overeating.

- Skullcap tea. This is excellent for headaches due to nervous tension.

Name: .... Date: ....

Symptoms and questions (be as specific as possible): ....

....

....

....

HEALTH-CARE VISIT

Practitioner consulted: ....

Tests and screening procedures performed, if any:

      Test (specify) ....

      Result ....

      Test (specify) ....

      Result ....

      Test (specify) ....

      Result ....

Treatments administered during the visit, if any: ....

....

Practitioner's observations/recommendations/answers to questions: ....

....

....

TREATMENTS USED

Conventional medicine: .... Responses and observations: ....

....

Herbal medicine: .... Responses and observations: ....

....

Homeopathic medicine: .... Responses and observations: ....

....

Diet/nutritional supplements: .... Responses and observations: ....

....

Other treatments/measures: .... Responses and observations: ....

....

Follow-up Questions and Observations ....

....

....

Name: .... Date: ....

Symptoms and questions (be as specific as possible):
....
....
....

HEALTH-CARE VISIT

Practitioner consulted: ....

Tests and screening procedures performed, if any:

Test (specify) ....

Result ....

Test (specify) ....

Result ....

Test (specify) ....

Result ....

Treatments administered during the visit, if any:
....

Practitioner's observations/recommendations/answers to questions:
....
....

TREATMENTS USED

Conventional medicine: ....   Responses and observations: ....
....

Herbal medicine: ....   Responses and observations: ....
....

Homeopathic medicine: ....   Responses and observations: ....
....

Diet/nutritional supplements: ....   Responses and observations: ....
....

Other treatments/measures: ....   Responses and observations: ....
....

Follow-up Questions and Observations
....
....

Name: .... Date: ....

Symptoms and questions (be as specific as possible): ....
....
....

HEALTH-CARE VISIT

Practitioner consulted: ....

Tests and screening procedures performed, if any:

Test (specify) ....

Result ....

Test (specify) ....

Result ....

Test (specify) ....

Result ....

Treatments administered during the visit, if any: ....

Practitioner's observations/recommendations/answers to questions: ....
....

Health Spotlight: Cold Sores

Cold sores are not actually caused by colds, but by the herpes simplex virus. This common name for those annoying sores probably comes from the fact that a herpes-related outbreak is more likely if a person's immune system is under stress, such as when fighting off infection, and a cold is the most common type of infection. Other infectious illnesses, allergies, emotional stress, and even exposure to sun and wind can lead to outbreaks just as well as colds can.

Canker sores look very much like cold sores. However, canker sores are small, swollen, painful ulcers, whereas cold sores start as small, irritating fluid-filled blisters that turn into red, burning, itchy sores. Also, cold sores usually occur on the hard part of the gums or on the "dry" part of the lips (and in exactly the same place every time), while canker sores occur on the "loose" part of the gums, the insides of the cheeks, or the inner lip.

One simple but effective home remedy for the discomfort of cold sores is to wet an ordinary black tea bag and place it on the open sores for five to ten minutes several times a day.

TREATMENTS USED

Conventional medicine: .... Responses and observations: ....

Herbal medicine: .... Responses and observations: ....

Homeopathic medicine: .... Responses and observations: ....

Diet/nutritional supplements: .... Responses and observations: ....

Other treatments/measures: .... Responses and observations: ....

Follow-up Questions and Observations ....

Name: .... Date: ....

Symptoms and questions (be as specific as possible): ....

....

....

HEALTH-CARE VISIT

Practitioner consulted: ....

Tests and screening procedures performed, if any:

    Test (specify) ....

    Result ....

    Test (specify) ....

    Result ....

    Test (specify) ....

    Result ....

Treatments administered during the visit, if any: ....

....

Practitioner's observations/recommendations/answers to questions: ....

....

....

TREATMENTS USED

Conventional medicine:	Responses and observations:
Herbal medicine:	Responses and observations:
Homeopathic medicine:	Responses and observations:
Diet/nutritional supplements:	Responses and observations:
Other treatments/measures:	Responses and observations:

Follow-up Questions and Observations ....

....

....

....

Name: .... Date: ....
Symptoms and questions (be as specific as possible):
....
....
....

HEALTH-CARE VISIT

Practitioner consulted: ....
Tests and screening procedures performed, if any:
    Test (specify) ....
    Result ....
    Test (specify) ....
    Result ....
    Test (specify) ....
    Result ....
Treatments administered during the visit, if any:
....
Practitioner's observations/recommendations/answers to questions:
....
....
....

TREATMENTS USED

Conventional medicine: .... Responses and observations: ....
....

Herbal medicine: .... Responses and observations: ....
....

Homeopathic medicine: .... Responses and observations: ....
....

Diet/nutritional supplements: .... Responses and observations: ....
....

Other treatments/measures: .... Responses and observations: ....
....
....

Follow-up Questions and Observations ....
....
....

Name: .... Date: ....

Symptoms and questions (be as specific as possible): ....

....

....

HEALTH-CARE VISIT

Practitioner consulted: ....

Tests and screening procedures performed, if any:

    Test (specify) ....

    Result ....

    Test (specify) ....

    Result ....

    Test (specify) ....

    Result ....

Treatments administered during the visit, if any: ....

....

Practitioner's observations/recommendations/answers to questions: ....

....

....

TREATMENTS USED

Conventional medicine: ....   Responses and observations: ....

....

Herbal medicine: ....   Responses and observations: ....

....

Homeopathic medicine: ....   Responses and observations: ....

....

Diet/nutritional supplements: ....   Responses and observations: ....

....

Other treatments/measures: ....   Responses and observations: ....

....

Follow-up Questions and Observations ....

....

....

Name: .... Date: ....

Symptoms and questions (be as specific as possible):
....
....
....

Health Spotlight: Stopping Hiccups

Hiccups are usually harmless and most go away on their own within a few minutes. If you'd rather not wait, try one of the following techniques:

- Slowly sip several glasses of cold water.

- Take a deep breath and hold it for as long as possible. It may help if you tip your head far backward while doing this.

- Breathe into a paper bag.

- Slowly sip cold water while holding your breath.

- Gargle with water for a minute or two.

- Lean over and sip cold water from the opposite rim of the glass.

- Have someone close your ears with his or her thumbs and slowly sip water while holding your breath.

- Try pulling on your tongue, pressing gently on your eyeballs, or rapidly swallowing cold water or small bits of ice. These measures stimulate the vagus nerve, which can help stop hiccups.

HEALTH-CARE VISIT

Practitioner consulted: ....

Tests and screening procedures performed, if any:

Test (specify) ....

Result ....

Test (specify) ....

Result ....

Test (specify) ....

Result ....

Treatments administered during the visit, if any:
....
....

Practitioner's observations/recommendations/answers to questions:
....
....

TREATMENTS USED

Conventional medicine:	Responses and observations:
Herbal medicine:	Responses and observations:
Homeopathic medicine:	Responses and observations:
Diet/nutritional supplements:	Responses and observations:
Other treatments/measures:	Responses and observations:

Follow-up Questions and Observations
....
....

Name: .... Date: ....

Symptoms and questions (be as specific as possible):
....
....
....

HEALTH-CARE VISIT

Practitioner consulted: ....

Tests and screening procedures performed, if any:

    Test (specify) ....

    Result ....

    Test (specify) ....

    Result ....

    Test (specify) ....

    Result ....

Treatments administered during the visit, if any:
....

Practitioner's observations/recommendations/answers to questions:
....
....

TREATMENTS USED

Conventional medicine:	Responses and observations:
....	....
....	....
Herbal medicine:	Responses and observations:
....	....
....	....
Homeopathic medicine:	Responses and observations:
....	....
....	....
Diet/nutritional supplements:	Responses and observations:
....	....
....	....
Other treatments/measures:	Responses and observations:
....	....
....	....

Follow-up Questions and Observations
....
....
....

Name: .... Date: ....

Symptoms and questions (be as specific as possible): ....
....
....

HEALTH-CARE VISIT

Practitioner consulted: ....

Tests and screening procedures performed, if any:

    Test (specify) ....

    Result ....

    Test (specify) ....

    Result ....

    Test (specify) ....

    Result ....

Treatments administered during the visit, if any: ....
....

Practitioner's observations/recommendations/answers to questions: ....
....
....

TREATMENTS USED

Conventional medicine:	Responses and observations:
Herbal medicine:	Responses and observations:
Homeopathic medicine:	Responses and observations:
Diet/nutritional supplements:	Responses and observations:
Other treatments/measures:	Responses and observations:

Follow-up Questions and Observations ....
....
....

Name: .... Date: ....

Symptoms and questions (be as specific as possible): ....

....

....

HEALTH-CARE VISIT

Practitioner consulted: ....

Tests and screening procedures performed, if any:

    Test (specify) ....

    Result ....

    Test (specify) ....

    Result ....

    Test (specify) ....

    Result ....

Treatments administered during the visit, if any: ....

....

Practitioner's observations/recommendations/answers to questions: ....

....

TREATMENTS USED

Conventional medicine:	Responses and observations:
Herbal medicine:	Responses and observations:
Homeopathic medicine:	Responses and observations:
Diet/nutritional supplements:	Responses and observations:
Other treatments/measures:	Responses and observations:

Follow-up Questions and Observations

....

....

Health Spotlight: Acne

According to *The Journal of the American Academy of Dermatology:*

- About 85 percent of the American population develops acne at some point during the teenage years.

- Acne can occur in children as young as six or seven years old.

- The peak incidence for acne in girls is between fourteen and seventeen years old.

- For boys, the incidence of acne is highest between the ages of sixteen and nineteen years.

- Most cases of teenage acne are benign and self-limiting, and are fully resolved by the time a person reaches his or her twenties.

Name: ....   Date: ....

Symptoms and questions (be as specific as possible): ....

....

....

Health Spotlight: Blood Pressure

- Blood pressure is the force exerted by the blood against arterial walls. It is what keeps the blood circulating.

- The first number in a blood-pressure measurement is the systolic pressure (pressure at the moment the heart beats). The second is the diastolic pressure (pressure between beats, when the heart is relaxed).

- There is no single blood-pressure reading that is normal for everyone. Most newborns have systolic readings between 20 and 60, and that number generally rises progressively throughout life. For healthy adults, a reading of 120/80 (120 over 80) is widely considered the norm, although blood pressure normally rises somewhat with age and actually varies throughout the day in response to the level of activity, stress, and other factors.

HEALTH-CARE VISIT

Practitioner consulted: ....

Tests and screening procedures performed, if any:

Test (specify) ....

Result ....

Test (specify) ....

Result ....

Test (specify) ....

Result ....

Treatments administered during the visit, if any:

....

Practitioner's observations/recommendations/answers to questions:

....

....

TREATMENTS USED

Conventional medicine: ....   Responses and observations: ....

....

....

Herbal medicine: ....   Responses and observations: ....

....

....

Homeopathic medicine: ....   Responses and observations: ....

....

....

....

Diet/nutritional supplements: ....   Responses and observations: ....

....

....

Other treatments/measures: ....   Responses and observations: ....

....

....

....

Follow-up Questions and Observations

....

....

....

Name: .... Date: ....

Symptoms and questions (be as specific as possible): ....

....

....

HEALTH-CARE VISIT

Practitioner consulted: ....

Tests and screening procedures performed, if any:

    Test (specify) ....

    Result ....

    Test (specify) ....

    Result ....

    Test (specify) ....

    Result ....

Treatments administered during the visit, if any: ....

....

Practitioner's observations/recommendations/answers to questions: ....

....

TREATMENTS USED

Conventional medicine:	Responses and observations:
Herbal medicine:	Responses and observations:
Homeopathic medicine:	Responses and observations:
Diet/nutritional supplements:	Responses and observations:
Other treatments/measures:	Responses and observations:

Follow-up Questions and Observations

....

....

....

- Tense or excitable individuals often experience a rise in blood pressure simply as a result of having their blood pressure read, which results in a false reading. This is known as "white-coat" hypertension (high blood pressure).

- About 90 percent of all people diagnosed with elevated blood pressure suffer from essential, or primary, hypertension—high blood pressure that has no obvious underlying cause.

- It was once widely accepted that consuming too much sodium (salt) leads to high blood pressure. Scientists now know that this is true only for certain individuals. In general, a correct balance among a number of minerals—sodium, potassium, calcium, and magnesium, among others—is more important for maintaining normal blood pressure.

Name: .... Date: ....

Symptoms and questions (be as specific as possible): ....

....

....

HEALTH-CARE VISIT

Practitioner consulted: ....

Tests and screening procedures performed, if any: ....

Test (specify) ....

Result ....

Test (specify) ....

Result ....

Test (specify) ....

Result ....

Treatments administered during the visit, if any: ....

....

Practitioner's observations/recommendations/answers to questions: ....

....

....

Health Spotlight: Natural Sleep Promoters

Having trouble getting a good night's sleep? Try one or more of the following:

- Make sure your diet includes foods containing the amino acid tryptophan, such as bananas, cottage cheese, fish, dates, milk, peanuts, and turkey. Having complex carbohydrates such as pasta or rice for dinner is a good sleep-inducer, too. Avoid eating excessive carbohydrates for three hours before bedtime, however.

- Take a teaspoon of brewer's yeast and/or a combination calcium and magnesium supplement an hour before bedtime.

- Take a dose of homeopathic *Coffea cruda* one hour before dinner and another dose a half hour before bedtime.

TREATMENTS USED

Conventional medicine: .... Responses and observations: ....

....

Herbal medicine: .... Responses and observations: ....

....

Homeopathic medicine: .... Responses and observations: ....

....

Diet/nutritional supplements: .... Responses and observations: ....

....

Other treatments/measures: .... Responses and observations: ....

....

Follow-up Questions and Observations

....

....

....

Name: .... Date: ....

Symptoms and questions (be as specific as possible):

....

....

HEALTH-CARE VISIT

Practitioner consulted:

....

Tests and screening procedures performed, if any:

    Test (specify) ....

    Result ....

    Test (specify) ....

    Result ....

    Test (specify) ....

    Result ....

Treatments administered during the visit, if any:

....

Practitioner's observations/recommendations/answers to questions:

....

TREATMENTS USED

Conventional medicine:	Responses and observations:
Herbal medicine:	Responses and observations:
Homeopathic medicine:	Responses and observations:
Diet/nutritional supplements:	Responses and observations:
Other treatments/measures:	Responses and observations:

Follow-up Questions and Observations

....

....

- Drink a cup of calming herbal tea before bed. Possibilities include chamomile, a chamomile combination such as Celestial Seasonings' Sleepytime, or a tea combining equal amounts of chamomile, passionflower, skullcap, and valerian.

- Have someone give you a back rub (focusing on the muscles on either side of the spine) or a foot rub shortly before you go to bed.

- Soak in a hot (102°F) bath for thirty minutes two hours before going to bed. For greater benefit, add several drops of essential oil of lavender, neroli, chamomile, or ylang ylang to the bathwater.

Name: .... Date: ....

Symptoms and questions (be as specific as possible): ....

....

....

HEALTH-CARE VISIT

Practitioner consulted: ....

Tests and screening procedures performed, if any:

    Test (specify) ....

    Result ....

    Test (specify) ....

    Result ....

    Test (specify) ....

    Result ....

Treatments administered during the visit, if any: ....

....

Practitioner's observations/recommendations/answers to questions: ....

....

....

TREATMENTS USED

Conventional medicine:	Responses and observations:
Herbal medicine:	Responses and observations:
Homeopathic medicine:	Responses and observations:
Diet/nutritional supplements:	Responses and observations:
Other treatments/measures:	Responses and observations:

Follow-up Questions and Observations

....

....

....

HEALTH SPOTLIGHT:
CAFFEINE CONTENT OF SELECTED FOODS
AND MEDICINES

It is estimated that 85 percent of Americans consume caffeine on a regular basis. While it is not considered harmful in reasonable quantities—indeed, there is even evidence that it can improve intellectual functioning and athletic stamina—it can be a problem for some people, causing jitteriness and contributing to insomnia. Use the table below to see how much caffeine you are consuming.

Food/Medicine (Quantity)	Caffeine Content
Chocolate:	
dark chocolate (1 ounce)	5–35 milligrams
milk chocolate (1 ounce)	1–10 milligrams
Chocolate cake (1 slice)	20–30 milligrams
Cocoa, hot (6 fluid ounces)	2–20 milligrams
Coffee:	
decaffeinated (6 fluid ounces)	2–7 milligrams
espresso (2 fluid ounces)	90–110 milligrams
regular, drip/brewed (6 fluid ounces)	80–175 milligrams
regular, instant (6 fluid ounces)	60–100 milligrams
Cola (12 fluid ounces)	45 milligrams
Tea:	
black (6 fluid ounces)	20–100 milligrams
green (6 fluid ounces)	20 milligrams
Anacin or Midol (2 tablets)	64 milligrams
Excedrin (2 tablets)	130 milligrams
NoDoz (2 tablets)	200 milligrams

Name: .... Date: ....

Symptoms and questions (be as specific as possible):

....

....

....

Health Spotlight: Lactose Intolerance

- Lactose is a type of sugar present in milk products. Digesting lactose requires the enzyme lactase. If you do not produce sufficient lactase, undigested lactose can ferment in the digestive system, causing bloating, cramping, abdominal gas, and diarrhea after you consume dairy products.

- Babies and young children almost always produce ample amounts of lactase, but starting at age six or seven, lactase production often begins to fall. In some people, it virtually disappears by adolescence.

- Lactose intolerance occurs in about 25 percent of Caucasians of northern European descent, but in 50 to 95 percent of people of other ethnic backgrounds.

- Some dairy products are more likely than others to provoke symptoms. Milk, cottage cheese, and ice cream usually cause more problems than aged cheeses or yogurt.

HEALTH-CARE VISIT

Practitioner consulted: ....

Tests and screening procedures performed, if any:

Test (specify) ....

Result ....

Test (specify) ....

Result ....

Test (specify) ....

Result ....

Treatments administered during the visit, if any:

....

....

Practitioner's observations/recommendations/answers to questions:

....

....

TREATMENTS USED

Conventional medicine:	Responses and observations:
Herbal medicine:	Responses and observations:
Homeopathic medicine:	Responses and observations:
Diet/nutritional supplements:	Responses and observations:
Other treatments/measures:	Responses and observations:

Follow-up Questions and Observations

....

....

....

Name: .... Date: ....

Symptoms and questions (be as specific as possible): ....

....

....

HEALTH-CARE VISIT

Practitioner consulted: ....

Tests and screening procedures performed, if any: ....

     Test (specify) ....

     Result ....

     Test (specify) ....

     Result ....

     Test (specify) ....

     Result ....

Treatments administered during the visit, if any: ....

....

Practitioner's observations/recommendations/answers to questions: ....

....

TREATMENTS USED

Conventional medicine:	Responses and observations:
Herbal medicine:	Responses and observations:
Homeopathic medicine:	Responses and observations:
Diet/nutritional supplements:	Responses and observations:
Other treatments/measures:	Responses and observations:

Follow-up Questions and Observations ....

....

....

Name: .... Date: ....

Symptoms and questions (be as specific as possible):

....

....

HEALTH-CARE VISIT

Health Spotlight: Motion Sickness

Practitioner consulted:

....

Tests and screening procedures performed, if any:

- Motion sickness occurs because abnormal or irregular body motions or postures, as well as repeated acceleration and deceleration, disturb the delicate balance mechanisms in the inner ear. Contradictory visual cues, which can occur when the body is passive but the landscape is rushing by, also play a part.

    Test (specify) ....

    Result ....

    Test (specify) ....

    Result ....

    Test (specify) ....

    Result ....

- Motion sickness is easier to prevent than it is to cure. In fact, relief usually does not occur right away once motion stops. It can take several hours for the body to recover, even after the trip is over.

Treatments administered during the visit, if any:

....

Practitioner's observations/recommendations/answers to questions:

....

....

- If you are prone to motion sickness, investigate whether you travel better on a full or empty stomach, and plan accordingly.

TREATMENTS USED

Conventional medicine:	Responses and observations:

- Try using Ear Planes. These are special earplugs that maintain even air pressure within the ears. The same effect may be achieved by holding foam drinking cups very tightly over each ear.

Herbal medicine:	Responses and observations:

Homeopathic medicine:	Responses and observations:

Diet/nutritional supplements:	Responses and observations:

Other treatments/measures:	Responses and observations:

Follow-up Questions and Observations

....

....

....

Name: .... Date: ....

Symptoms and questions (be as specific as possible): ....

....

....

HEALTH-CARE VISIT

Practitioner consulted: ....

Tests and screening procedures performed, if any:

    Test (specify) ....

    Result ....

    Test (specify) ....

    Result ....

    Test (specify) ....

    Result ....

Treatments administered during the visit, if any: ....

....

Practitioner's observations/recommendations/answers to questions: ....

....

TREATMENTS USED

Conventional medicine: ....

....

....

Herbal medicine: ....

....

....

Homeopathic medicine: ....

....

....

Diet/nutritional supplements: ....

....

....

Other treatments/measures: ....

....

....

Responses and observations: ....

....

....

Responses and observations: ....

....

....

Responses and observations: ....

....

....

Responses and observations: ....

....

....

Responses and observations: ....

....

....

Follow-up Questions and Observations ....

....

....

- Learn to hold your head very still while traveling. Focus your eyes on a fixed point on the far-distant horizon.

- Open a window or direct a vent to blow cool air across your face.

- Avoid reading while in a moving vehicle.

- Carry a thermos of warm or room-temperature ginger tea with you and sip it as needed.

- Homeopathic remedies can be helpful. Again, observe your symptoms closely and choose the appropriate remedy accordingly. *Cocculus* should help if you feel nauseated, if the smell of food makes you feel sick, and if you feel better under warm blankets. If you feel better after eating, when resting quietly with your eyes closed, and when you know the trip will soon be over, take homeopathic *Petroleum*. If you are pale, in a cold sweat, feel faint, and are nauseated and vomiting, try *Tabacum*.

HEALTH SPOTLIGHT:
SPRAINED ANKLES

- The most commonly sprained joint is the ankle. More than 20,000 ankle sprains occur each day in the United States.
- Most sprained ankles are caused by the twisting of an ankle.
- About 85 percent of ankle sprains are inversion sprains, in which the foot twists inward and the outside ligaments are stretched or torn.
- About 15 percent of ankle sprains are eversion sprains, in which the foot twists outward, causing damage to the ligaments on the inner side of the ankle.
- Ankle sprains are divided into three classes, depending on severity, as described in the table below.

Type of Sprain	Description	Time to Full Recovery
First-degree	Stretching and minimal tearing, pain, tenderness, and swelling, but no bruising or loss of function.	4–6 weeks
Second-degree	A tearing sensation, pop, or snap, gradually developing swelling, tenderness, and bruising. Walking may be difficult.	4–8 weeks
Third-degree	The joint may slip out of place, then back in, with massive swelling, severe tenderness, and instability. Walking may be impossible.	6–12 weeks

Name: .... Date: ....

Symptoms and questions (be as specific as possible): ....

....

....

....

HEALTH-CARE VISIT

Practitioner consulted: ....

Tests and screening procedures performed, if any: ....

    Test (specify) ....

    Result ....

    Test (specify) ....

    Result ....

    Test (specify) ....

    Result ....

Treatments administered during the visit, if any: ....

....

Practitioner's observations/recommendations/answers to questions: ....

....

....

TREATMENTS USED

Conventional medicine: ....   Responses and observations: ....

....

Herbal medicine: ....   Responses and observations: ....

....

Homeopathic medicine: ....   Responses and observations: ....

....

Diet/nutritional supplements: ....   Responses and observations: ....

....

Other treatments/measures: ....   Responses and observations: ....

....

Follow-up Questions and Observations ....

....

....

Name: .... Date: ....

Symptoms and questions (be as specific as possible):

....

....

....

Health Spotlight: Finger- and Toenail Conditions

There are many different health problems that can affect the condition of the nails, including the following:

- Blackish, splinterlike bits in the nails can be a sign of bacterial endocarditis, a heart infection.

- Easily broken nails can be a sign of deficiency of calcium, silica, and/or certain other trace minerals.

- Horizontal ridges can be an indicator of injury, infection, or illness.

- Pitted nails may be associated with psoriasis.

- Spoon-shaped nails are associated with iron deficiency.

- Vertical ridges in the nails may point to poor absorption of nutrients.

- Very pale-colored nail beds may be a sign of anemia.

- White spots in the nails may signify a zinc deficiency.

If you develop any of these conditions, you may wish to bring it to the attention of a health-care professional.

HEALTH-CARE VISIT

Practitioner consulted: ....

Tests and screening procedures performed, if any:

    Test (specify) ....

    Result ....

    Test (specify) ....

    Result ....

    Test (specify) ....

    Result ....

Treatments administered during the visit, if any:

....

Practitioner's observations/recommendations/answers to questions:

....

TREATMENTS USED

Conventional medicine:	Responses and observations:
Herbal medicine:	Responses and observations:
Homeopathic medicine:	Responses and observations:
Diet/nutritional supplements:	Responses and observations:
Other treatments/measures:	Responses and observations:

Follow-up Questions and Observations

....

....

....

Name: .... Date: ....

Symptoms and questions (be as specific as possible): ....
....
....

HEALTH-CARE VISIT

Practitioner consulted: ....

Tests and screening procedures performed, if any:

    Test (specify) ....

    Result ....

    Test (specify) ....

    Result ....

    Test (specify) ....

    Result ....

Treatments administered during the visit, if any: ....
....

Practitioner's observations/recommendations/answers to questions: ....
....
....

TREATMENTS USED

Conventional medicine:	Responses and observations: ....
....	....
Herbal medicine:	Responses and observations: ....
....	....
Homeopathic medicine:	Responses and observations: ....
....	....
Diet/nutritional supplements:	Responses and observations: ....
....	....
Other treatments/measures:	Responses and observations: ....
....	....

Follow-up Questions and Observations
....
....
....

Name: .... Date: ....

Symptoms and questions (be as specific as possible): ....

....

....

HEALTH-CARE VISIT

Practitioner consulted: ....

Tests and screening procedures performed, if any:

Test (specify) ....

Result ....

Test (specify) ....

Result ....

Test (specify) ....

Result ....

Treatments administered during the visit, if any: ....

....

Practitioner's observations/recommendations/answers to questions: ....

....

....

TREATMENTS USED

Conventional medicine: .... Responses and observations: ....

....

Herbal medicine: .... Responses and observations: ....

....

Homeopathic medicine: .... Responses and observations: ....

....

Diet/nutritional supplements: .... Responses and observations: ....

....

Other treatments/measures: .... Responses and observations: ....

....

Follow-up Questions and Observations

....

....

....

Name: .... Date: ....

Symptoms and questions (be as specific as possible): ....

....

....

HEALTH-CARE VISIT

Practitioner consulted: ....

Tests and screening procedures performed, if any:

    Test (specify) ....

    Result ....

    Test (specify) ....

    Result ....

    Test (specify) ....

    Result ....

Treatments administered during the visit, if any: ....

....

Practitioner's observations/recommendations/answers to questions: ....

....

....

TREATMENTS USED

Conventional medicine:	Responses and observations:
Herbal medicine:	Responses and observations:
Homeopathic medicine:	Responses and observations:
Diet/nutritional supplements:	Responses and observations:
Other treatments/measures:	Responses and observations:

Follow-up Questions and Observations ....

....

....

Health Spotlight: How to Stop a Nosebleed

1. Calmly sit down in an upright position, not leaning back. Breathe through your mouth.

2. Tilt your head forward (*not* backward).

3. Place your thumb and forefinger on either side of the bridge of your nose and pinch the soft part of your nose firmly for ten minutes without releasing. Apply pressure firmly enough to slow bleeding, but not so strongly as to cause discomfort.

4. After ten minutes, release the nostrils slowly and check to see if the bleeding has stopped. Avoid touching or blowing your nose. If the bleeding has not stopped, apply pressure for another ten-minute period.

5. If your nose is still bleeding steadily after twenty minutes of pressure, call your health-care provider.

Another way to stop a nosebleed is to wet a bit of cotton or plain sterile gauze with white vinegar, place it in your nose, and leave it in place for at least ten minutes.

Name: .... Date: ....

Symptoms and questions (be as specific as possible): ....

....

....

HEALTH-CARE VISIT

Practitioner consulted: ....

Tests and screening procedures performed, if any:

    Test (specify) ....

    Result ....

    Test (specify) ....

    Result ....

    Test (specify) ....

    Result ....

Treatments administered during the visit, if any: ....

....

Practitioner's observations/recommendations/answers to questions: ....

....

....

TREATMENTS USED

Conventional medicine:	Responses and observations:
Herbal medicine:	Responses and observations:
Homeopathic medicine:	Responses and observations:
Diet/nutritional supplements:	Responses and observations:
Other treatments/measures:	Responses and observations:

Follow-up Questions and Observations

....

....

....

HEALTH SPOTLIGHT:
CALCIUM CONTENT OF SELECTED FOODS

Calcium is a vital mineral for many body functions, among them proper muscle (including heart muscle) contraction and the formation of bone. Refer to the following table to see how much calcium you're getting in the foods you eat.

Food (Quantity)	Calcium Content
Bread (1 slice)	20–40 milligrams
Broccoli, cooked (1 cup)	90 milligrams
Cheddar cheese (1 ounces)	205 milligrams
Cottage cheese (8 ounces)	150 milligrams
Ice cream/ice milk (8 ounces)	175 milligrams
Kale, cooked (1 cup)	95 milligrams
Milk (8 fluid ounces)	300 milligrams
Orange juice, calcium-fortified (8 fluid ounces)	300 milligrams
Salmon, with bones (3 ounces)	225 milligrams
Sardines, with bones (3 ounces)	370 milligrams
Swiss cheese (1 ounce)	270 milligrams
Tofu (2 ounces)	115 milligrams
Turnip greens, cooked (1 cup)	200 milligrams
Yogurt, fruit-flavored (8 ounces)	300 milligrams
Yogurt, plain, nonfat (8 ounces)	450 milligrams

Name: .... Date: ....

Symptoms and questions (be as specific as possible): ....

....

....

HEALTH-CARE VISIT

Practitioner consulted: ....

Tests and screening procedures performed, if any:

    Test (specify) ....

    Result ....

    Test (specify) ....

    Result ....

    Test (specify) ....

    Result ....

Treatments administered during the visit, if any: ....

....

Practitioner's observations/recommendations/answers to questions: ....

....

....

TREATMENTS USED

Conventional medicine:	Responses and observations:
Herbal medicine:	Responses and observations:
Homeopathic medicine:	Responses and observations:
Diet/nutritional supplements:	Responses and observations:
Other treatments/measures:	Responses and observations:

Follow-up Questions and Observations ....

....

....

Name: ....   Date: ....

Symptoms and questions (be as specific as possible): ....

....

....

HEALTH-CARE VISIT

Practitioner consulted: ....

Tests and screening procedures performed, if any:

    Test (specify) ....

    Result ....

    Test (specify) ....

    Result ....

    Test (specify) ....

    Result ....

Treatments administered during the visit, if any: ....

....

Practitioner's observations/recommendations/answers to questions: ....

....

....

TREATMENTS USED

Conventional medicine:	Responses and observations:
Herbal medicine:	Responses and observations:
Homeopathic medicine:	Responses and observations:
Diet/nutritional supplements:	Responses and observations:
Other treatments/measures:	Responses and observations:

Follow-up Questions and Observations ....

....

....

Name: .... Date: ....

Symptoms and questions (be as specific as possible): ....

....

....

HEALTH-CARE VISIT

Health Spotlight: Pain-Relief Tea

To make a gentle herbal pain-relief tea, do the following:

1. Simmer 1 tablespoon of white willow bark* in 1 quart of water for fifteen minutes.

2. Add 1 tablespoon of chamomile, 1 tablespoon of skullcap, 1 tablespoon of valerian root, and ½ tablespoon of licorice root.* Simmer for another ten minutes.

3. Remove from heat, strain, and cool.

To help relieve generalized pain, take a cup every hour for four consecutive hours. White willow bark is an anti-inflammatory similar to aspirin; chamomile is an effective relaxant; skullcap and valerian have sedative and antispasmodic properties; and licorice is an anti-inflammatory and enhances the action of the other herbs, in addition to sweetening the tea.

*Do not use licorice on a daily basis for more than five days at a time, however, as it can elevate blood pressure. Do not use white willow bark if you are allergic to aspirin or taking a blood thinner such as coumadin, and do not give it to a child except at the direction of a health-care professional.

Practitioner consulted: ....

Tests and screening procedures performed, if any:

Test (specify) ....

Result ....

Test (specify) ....

Result ....

Test (specify) ....

Result ....

Treatments administered during the visit, if any:

....

Practitioner's observations/recommendations/answers to questions: ....

....

TREATMENTS USED

Conventional medicine: ....

Responses and observations: ....

Herbal medicine: ....

Responses and observations: ....

Homeopathic medicine: ....

Responses and observations: ....

Diet/nutritional supplements: ....

Responses and observations: ....

Other treatments/measures: ....

Responses and observations: ....

Follow-up Questions and Observations

....

....

....

Name: .... Date: ....

Symptoms and questions (be as specific as possible): ....

....

....

HEALTH-CARE VISIT

Practitioner consulted: ....

Tests and screening procedures performed, if any:

    Test (specify) ....

    Result ....

    Test (specify) ....

    Result ....

    Test (specify) ....

    Result ....

Treatments administered during the visit, if any: ....

....

Practitioner's observations/recommendations/answers to questions: ....

....

....

TREATMENTS USED

Conventional medicine:	Responses and observations:
....	....
....	....
Herbal medicine:	Responses and observations:
....	....
....	....
Homeopathic medicine:	Responses and observations:
....	....
....	....
Diet/nutritional supplements:	Responses and observations:
....	....
....	....
Other treatments/measures:	Responses and observations:
....	....
....	....

Follow-up Questions and Observations ....

....

....

Name: .... Date: ....

Symptoms and questions (be as specific as possible): ....

....

....

HEALTH-CARE VISIT

Practitioner consulted: ....

Tests and screening procedures performed, if any:

    Test (specify) ....

    Result ....

    Test (specify) ....

    Result ....

    Test (specify) ....

    Result ....

Treatments administered during the visit, if any: ....

....

Practitioner's observations/recommendations/answers to questions: ....

....

....

TREATMENTS USED

Conventional medicine:	Responses and observations:
Herbal medicine:	Responses and observations:
Homeopathic medicine:	Responses and observations:
Diet/nutritional supplements:	Responses and observations:
Other treatments/measures:	Responses and observations:

Follow-up Questions and Observations ....

....

....

Name: _____   Date: _____

Symptoms and questions (be as specific as possible):

....

....

HEALTH-CARE VISIT

Practitioner consulted: _____

Tests and screening procedures performed, if any:

    Test (specify) _____

    Result _____

    Test (specify) _____

    Result _____

    Test (specify) _____

    Result _____

Treatments administered during the visit, if any:

....

Practitioner's observations/recommendations/answers to questions:

....

TREATMENTS USED

Conventional medicine:	Responses and observations:
Herbal medicine:	Responses and observations:
Homeopathic medicine:	Responses and observations:
Diet/nutritional supplements:	Responses and observations:
Other treatments/measures:	Responses and observations:

Follow-up Questions and Observations

....

....

....

Health Spotlight:
Restless Legs Syndrome

- Restless legs syndrome (RLS) is a neurological condition characterized by sensations in the legs that can be difficult to describe, but have been characterized as twitching, tugging, crawling, tingling, itching, pulling, and burning.

- Symptoms occur most often in the evening and at night, but can also occur at other times.

- Despite the name, RLS symptoms may affect the arms as well as the legs.

- RLS is usually diagnosed in people between the ages of fifty and sixty, but it usually begins much earlier. Many recall having been scolded as children because they wouldn't sit still due to the discomfort. It is likely that many people who have RLS do not realize that their symptoms actually have a name.

- The cause of RLS is not understood, but it is believed to be related to a problem in the nervous system that originates in either the brain or the spinal cord.

- Most people who have RLS can be helped with a combination of drug therapies and natural treatments including acupuncture.

Name: .... Date: ....

Symptoms and questions (be as specific as possible): ....

....

....

HEALTH-CARE VISIT

Practitioner consulted: ....

Tests and screening procedures performed, if any:

      Test (specify) ....

      Result ....

      Test (specify) ....

      Result ....

      Test (specify) ....

      Result ....

Treatments administered during the visit, if any: ....

....

Practitioner's observations/recommendations/answers to questions: ....

....

....

TREATMENTS USED

Conventional medicine:	Responses and observations:
Herbal medicine:	Responses and observations:
Homeopathic medicine:	Responses and observations:
Diet/nutritional supplements:	Responses and observations:
Other treatments/measures:	Responses and observations:

Follow-up Questions and Observations ....

....

....

Name: .... Date: ....

Symptoms and questions (be as specific as possible): ....

....

....

HEALTH-CARE VISIT

Practitioner consulted: ....

Tests and screening procedures performed, if any:

Test (specify) ....

Result ....

Test (specify) ....

Result ....

Test (specify) ....

Result ....

Treatments administered during the visit, if any: ....

....

Practitioner's observations/recommendations/answers to questions: ....

....

....

TREATMENTS USED

Conventional medicine: ....   Responses and observations: ....

....

Herbal medicine: ....   Responses and observations: ....

....

Homeopathic medicine: ....   Responses and observations: ....

....

Diet/nutritional supplements: ....   Responses and observations: ....

....

Other treatments/measures: ....   Responses and observations: ....

....

Follow-up Questions and Observations

....

....

....

Name: .... Date: ....

Symptoms and questions (be as specific as possible): ....

....

....

HEALTH-CARE VISIT

Health Spotlight: Natural Congestion Clearers

If you are suffering from a cold, the flu, a sinus infection, or any other congestion-causing disorder, try one or more of the following:

- Drink plenty of pure spring water.

- Eat chicken soup made with lots of vegetables. Medical science has confirmed what your mother always knew: Hot chicken soup with vegetables contains substances that promote healing and sinus drainage.

- Mix the juice of two freshly squeezed lemons with an equal amount of water and sweeten with a bit of maple syrup. If you can tolerate it, add ⅛ teaspoon of cayenne pepper.

- Make an herbal tea combining 1 tablespoon of fenugreek, 1 tablespoon of rose hips, 1 tablespoon of thyme, and ½ tablespoon of licorice brewed in 8 ounces of water. Take one cup twice a day. (Note: If you have high blood pressure, omit the licorice.)

Practitioner consulted: ....

Tests and screening procedures performed, if any: ....

    Test (specify) ....

    Result ....

    Test (specify) ....

    Result ....

    Test (specify) ....

    Result ....

Treatments administered during the visit, if any: ....

....

Practitioner's observations/recommendations/answers to questions: ....

....

TREATMENTS USED

Conventional medicine:	Responses and observations:
Herbal medicine:	Responses and observations:
Homeopathic medicine:	Responses and observations:
Diet/nutritional supplements:	Responses and observations:
Other treatments/measures:	Responses and observations:

Follow-up Questions and Observations

....

....

....

Name: .... Date: ....

Symptoms and questions (be as specific as possible):
....
....
....

HEALTH-CARE VISIT

Practitioner consulted:
....

Tests and screening procedures performed, if any:

    Test (specify) ....

    Result ....

    Test (specify) ....

    Result ....

    Test (specify) ....

    Result ....

Treatments administered during the visit, if any:
....

Practitioner's observations/recommendations/answers to questions:
....
....

- Grate a large ginger root into a pot containing 1 pint of water and simmer for fifteen minutes. Use the resulting tea to make a hot compress and place the compress over the sinus area.

- Make a rosemary steam inhalation by boiling a large pot of water with 1 tablespoon of rosemary for each quart of water. Place the pot on a table and position your head over the pot to inhale the steam. If possible, use a large towel to make a "tent" over your head to hold in the steam.

TREATMENTS USED

Conventional medicine:	Responses and observations:

Herbal medicine:	Responses and observations:

Homeopathic medicine:	Responses and observations:

Diet/nutritional supplements:	Responses and observations:

Other treatments/measures:	Responses and observations:

Follow-up Questions and Observations
....
....
....

Name:

Date:

Symptoms and questions (be as specific as possible):

HEALTH-CARE VISIT

Practitioner consulted:

Tests and screening procedures performed, if any:

Test (specify)

Result

Test (specify)

Result

Test (specify)

Result

Treatments administered during the visit, if any:

Practitioner's observations/recommendations/answers to questions:

TREATMENTS USED

Conventional medicine:

Responses and observations:

Herbal medicine:

Responses and observations:

Homeopathic medicine:

Responses and observations:

Diet/nutritional supplements:

Responses and observations:

Other treatments/measures:

Responses and observations:

Follow-up Questions and Observations

Name: .... Date: ....

Symptoms and questions (be as specific as possible):
....

....

....

HEALTH-CARE VISIT

Practitioner consulted: ....

Tests and screening procedures performed, if any:

    Test (specify) ....

    Result ....

    Test (specify) ....

    Result ....

    Test (specify) ....

    Result ....

Treatments administered during the visit, if any:
....

Practitioner's observations/recommendations/answers to questions:
....

....

Health Spotlight: Quick Relief for Skin Rashes

Regardless of the cause, if you develop a skin rash that is itchy and/or inflamed, cool compresses can often provide quick relief. Soak a clean cloth in cool water, wring it out, and apply it to the affected area for ten minutes. Repeat as often as necessary.

TREATMENTS USED

Conventional medicine: Responses and observations:

Herbal medicine: Responses and observations:

Homeopathic medicine: Responses and observations:

Diet/nutritional supplements: Responses and observations:

Other treatments/measures: Responses and observations:

Follow-up Questions and Observations
....

....

Name: .... Date: ....

Symptoms and questions (be as specific as possible): ....

....

....

HEALTH-CARE VISIT

Practitioner consulted: ....

Tests and screening procedures performed, if any:

     Test (specify) ....

     Result ....

     Test (specify) ....

     Result ....

     Test (specify) ....

     Result ....

Treatments administered during the visit, if any: ....

Practitioner's observations/recommendations/answers to questions: ....

....

....

TREATMENTS USED

Conventional medicine:	Responses and observations:
Herbal medicine:	Responses and observations:
Homeopathic medicine:	Responses and observations:
Diet/nutritional supplements:	Responses and observations:
Other treatments/measures:	Responses and observations:

Follow-up Questions and Observations ....

....

....

Name: .... Date: ....

Symptoms and questions (be as specific as possible): ....

....

....

HEALTH-CARE VISIT

Practitioner consulted: ....

Tests and screening procedures performed, if any:

Test (specify) ....

Result ....

Test (specify) ....

Result ....

Test (specify) ....

Result ....

Treatments administered during the visit, if any: ....

....

Practitioner's observations/recommendations/answers to questions: ....

....

TREATMENTS USED

Conventional medicine: .... Responses and observations: ....

Herbal medicine: .... Responses and observations: ....

Homeopathic medicine: .... Responses and observations: ....

Diet/nutritional supplements: .... Responses and observations: ....

Other treatments/measures: .... Responses and observations: ....

Follow-up Questions and Observations ....

....

Name: .... Date: ....

Symptoms and questions (be as specific as possible):

....

....

....

Health Spotlight: Snoring

- Snoring occurs when the uvula (the small, conical piece of flesh that projects downward from the soft palate in the middle of the mouth) vibrates.

- An estimated 40 million Americans snore.

- Almost twice as many men as women snore.

- Most people who snore sleep with their mouths open.

- Obesity increases the likelihood of snoring by a factor of three.

- You are much more likely to snore if you sleep on your back rather than on your side or stomach.

- Chronic snoring can be related to sleep apnea, which causes a person to stop breathing and then abruptly wake multiple times during the night, often without being aware of it. Sleep apnea can lead to daytime sleepiness and problems with concentration and memory. It also contributes to the risk of high blood pressure, cardiovascular problems, and stroke. The condition is usually treatable with a special breathing device, surgery, or medication.

- Homeopathic snore combination remedies can be very effective.

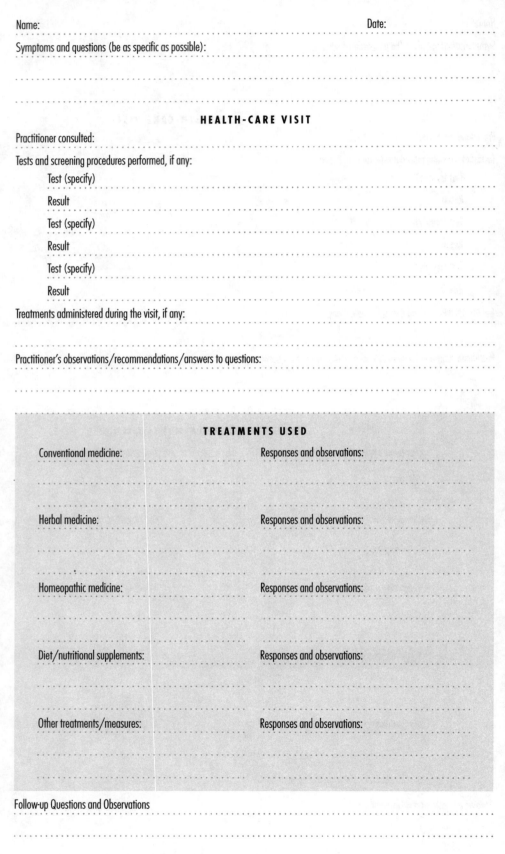

HEALTH-CARE VISIT

Practitioner consulted: ....

Tests and screening procedures performed, if any:

    Test (specify) ....

    Result ....

    Test (specify) ....

    Result ....

    Test (specify) ....

    Result ....

Treatments administered during the visit, if any:

....

Practitioner's observations/recommendations/answers to questions:

....

TREATMENTS USED

Conventional medicine: Responses and observations:

Herbal medicine: Responses and observations:

Homeopathic medicine: Responses and observations:

Diet/nutritional supplements: Responses and observations:

Other treatments/measures: Responses and observations:

Follow-up Questions and Observations

....

....

....

Name: .... Date: ....

Symptoms and questions (be as specific as possible): ....

....

....

HEALTH-CARE VISIT

Practitioner consulted: ....

Tests and screening procedures performed, if any:

    Test (specify) ....

    Result ....

    Test (specify) ....

    Result ....

    Test (specify) ....

    Result ....

Treatments administered during the visit, if any: ....

....

Practitioner's observations/recommendations/answers to questions: ....

....

....

TREATMENTS USED

Conventional medicine: ....   Responses and observations: ....

....

....

Herbal medicine: ....   Responses and observations: ....

....

....

Homeopathic medicine: ....   Responses and observations: ....

....

....

Diet/nutritional supplements: ....   Responses and observations: ....

....

....

Other treatments/measures: ....   Responses and observations: ....

....

....

Follow-up Questions and Observations ....

....

....

Name: .... Date: ....

Symptoms and questions (be as specific as possible): ....

....

....

HEALTH-CARE VISIT

Practitioner consulted: ....

Tests and screening procedures performed, if any:

    Test (specify) ....

    Result ....

    Test (specify) ....

    Result ....

    Test (specify) ....

    Result ....

Treatments administered during the visit, if any: ....

....

Practitioner's observations/recommendations/answers to questions: ....

....

....

TREATMENTS USED

Conventional medicine:	Responses and observations:
....	....
....	....
Herbal medicine:	Responses and observations:
....	....
....	....
Homeopathic medicine:	Responses and observations:
....	....
....	....
Diet/nutritional supplements:	Responses and observations:
....	....
....	....
Other treatments/measures:	Responses and observations:
....	....
....	....

Follow-up Questions and Observations

....

....

....

Name: .... Date: ....

Symptoms and questions (be as specific as possible): ....
....
....

HEALTH-CARE VISIT

Practitioner consulted: ....

Tests and screening procedures performed, if any:

    Test (specify) ....

    Result ....

    Test (specify) ....

    Result ....

    Test (specify) ....

    Result ....

Treatments administered during the visit, if any: ....
....

Practitioner's observations/recommendations/answers to questions: ....
....

TREATMENTS USED

Conventional medicine:	Responses and observations:
Herbal medicine:	Responses and observations:
Homeopathic medicine:	Responses and observations:
Diet/nutritional supplements:	Responses and observations:
Other treatments/measures:	Responses and observations:

Follow-up Questions and Observations
....
....

Health Spotlight: The RICE Technique

To prevent or minimize pain- and strain-type injury due to physical activity, use the RICE technique described below.

- Rest. If something you're doing hurts, stop and rest the affected area as soon as possible.

- Ice. Apply a cold compress by wrapping ice in a cloth and applying it to the affected area for twenty minutes, then remove the ice for twenty minutes. Repeat this over a period of a few hours or as needed.

- Compression. Wrap the area in an elastic bandage or strips of cloth, firmly enough to provide support and limit swelling, but not so tightly that you interfere with circulation. Compress the area for thirty minutes, then remove the compression for fifteen minutes to allow full circulation. Repeat this process over a period of a few hours or as needed.

- Elevation. Elevate the affected part to a level above your heart. Rest and relax for thirty minutes.

You can do these steps simultaneously or individually as the injury heals.

Name: .... Date: ....

Symptoms and questions (be as specific as possible): ....

....

....

HEALTH-CARE VISIT

Practitioner consulted: ....

Tests and screening procedures performed, if any:

    Test (specify) ....

    Result ....

    Test (specify) ....

    Result ....

    Test (specify) ....

    Result ....

Treatments administered during the visit, if any: ....

....

Practitioner's observations/recommendations/answers to questions: ....

....

TREATMENTS USED

Conventional medicine: .... Responses and observations: ....

....

Herbal medicine: .... Responses and observations: ....

....

Homeopathic medicine: .... Responses and observations: ....

....

Diet/nutritional supplements: .... Responses and observations: ....

....

Other treatments/measures: .... Responses and observations: ....

....

Follow-up Questions and Observations ....

....

....

Name: .... Date: ....

Symptoms and questions (be as specific as possible):

....

....

....

HEALTH-CARE VISIT

Practitioner consulted: ....

Tests and screening procedures performed, if any:

    Test (specify) ....

    Result ....

    Test (specify) ....

    Result ....

    Test (specify) ....

    Result ....

Treatments administered during the visit, if any:

....

Practitioner's observations/recommendations/answers to questions:

....

....

....

TREATMENTS USED

Conventional medicine: Responses and observations:

....

Herbal medicine: Responses and observations:

....

Homeopathic medicine: Responses and observations:

....

Diet/nutritional supplements: Responses and observations:

....

Other treatments/measures: Responses and observations:

....

Follow-up Questions and Observations

....

....

Name: .... Date: ....

Symptoms and questions (be as specific as possible): ....

....

....

HEALTH-CARE VISIT

Health Spotlight: Treating Warts with Banana Peels

A banana peel contains a substance that is highly effective at destroying warts. Many dermatologists recommend it. Place a small amount of peel against the wart and hold it in place with adhesive tape. Change the peel once or twice daily, as needed. Repeat for two weeks or until the wart is gone.

Practitioner consulted: ....

Tests and screening procedures performed, if any:

    Test (specify) ....

    Result ....

    Test (specify) ....

    Result ....

    Test (specify) ....

    Result ....

Treatments administered during the visit, if any: ....

....

Practitioner's observations/recommendations/answers to questions: ....

....

....

TREATMENTS USED

Conventional medicine: ....   Responses and observations: ....

....

Herbal medicine: ....   Responses and observations: ....

....

Homeopathic medicine: ....   Responses and observations: ....

....

Diet/nutritional supplements: ....   Responses and observations: ....

....

Other treatments/measures: ....   Responses and observations: ....

....

Follow-up Questions and Observations ....

....

....

Name: ....   Date: ....

Symptoms and questions (be as specific as possible): ....
....
....

HEALTH-CARE VISIT

Practitioner consulted: ....

Tests and screening procedures performed, if any:

Test (specify) ....

Result ....

Test (specify) ....

Result ....

Test (specify) ....

Result ....

Treatments administered during the visit, if any: ....
....

Practitioner's observations/recommendations/answers to questions: ....
....
....

TREATMENTS USED

Conventional medicine: ....   Responses and observations: ....
....
....

Herbal medicine: ....   Responses and observations: ....
....
....

Homeopathic medicine: ....   Responses and observations: ....
....
....

Diet/nutritional supplements: ....   Responses and observations: ....
....
....

Other treatments/measures: ....   Responses and observations: ....
....
....

Follow-up Questions and Observations ....
....
....

Name: .... Date: ....

Symptoms and questions (be as specific as possible): ....

....

....

HEALTH-CARE VISIT

Practitioner consulted: ....

Tests and screening procedures performed, if any: ....

    Test (specify) ....

    Result ....

    Test (specify) ....

    Result ....

    Test (specify) ....

    Result ....

Treatments administered during the visit, if any: ....

....

Practitioner's observations/recommendations/answers to questions: ....

....

....

TREATMENTS USED

Conventional medicine:	Responses and observations:
Herbal medicine:	Responses and observations:
Homeopathic medicine:	Responses and observations:
Diet/nutritional supplements:	Responses and observations:
Other treatments/measures:	Responses and observations:

Follow-up Questions and Observations ....

....

....

Name: .... Date: ....

Symptoms and questions (be as specific as possible): ....

....

....

HEALTH-CARE VISIT

Practitioner consulted: ....

Tests and screening procedures performed, if any:

Test (specify) ....

Result ....

Test (specify) ....

Result ....

Test (specify) ....

Result ....

Treatments administered during the visit, if any: ....

....

Practitioner's observations/recommendations/answers to questions: ....

....

....

TREATMENTS USED

Conventional medicine: .... | Responses and observations: ....

.... | ....

Herbal medicine: .... | Responses and observations: ....

.... | ....

Homeopathic medicine: .... | Responses and observations: ....

.... | ....

Diet/nutritional supplements: .... | Responses and observations: ....

.... | ....

Other treatments/measures: .... | Responses and observations: ....

.... | ....

.... | ....

Follow-up Questions and Observations

....

....

....

Name: ....   Date: ....

Symptoms and questions (be as specific as possible): ....
....
....

HEALTH-CARE VISIT

Health Spotlight: The Benefits of Exercise

Regular exercise is as vital as good nutrition for optimum health. The known benefits of exercise include the following:

- It leads to a reduction in blood pressure.

- It can prevent or help in overcoming obesity.

- It reduces levels of low-density lipoproteins (LDL, or "bad" cholesterol), while raising levels of high-density lipoproteins (HDL, or "good" cholesterol).

- It improves breathing and digestion.

- It helps to promote regular bowel habits.

- It is an excellent stress- and anxiety-reducer, and can even relieve the symptoms of more serious psychological conditions, including panic disorder and depression.

Practitioner consulted: ....

Tests and screening procedures performed, if any:

    Test (specify) ....

    Result ....

    Test (specify) ....

    Result ....

    Test (specify) ....

    Result ....

Treatments administered during the visit, if any:
....

Practitioner's observations/recommendations/answers to questions: ....
....

TREATMENTS USED

Conventional medicine:	Responses and observations:
Herbal medicine:	Responses and observations:
Homeopathic medicine:	Responses and observations:
Diet/nutritional supplements:	Responses and observations:
Other treatments/measures:	Responses and observations:

Follow-up Questions and Observations
....
....
....

Name: Date:

Symptoms and questions (be as specific as possible):

HEALTH-CARE VISIT

Practitioner consulted:

Tests and screening procedures performed, if any:

    Test (specify)

    Result

    Test (specify)

    Result

    Test (specify)

    Result

Treatments administered during the visit, if any:

Practitioner's observations/recommendations/answers to questions:

- It helps to maintain and improve the range of movement of important joints.

- It improves coordination and balance.

- It improves flexibility and strengthens muscles, thereby increasing endurance and stamina. Strengthening the muscles of the lower back and abdomen can help prevent or ease lower back pain.

- Weight-bearing exercise contributes to strong bones, which helps reduce the risk of osteoporosis.

Regular exercise is a habit best developed in childhood, but it is never too late to begin. A moderate degree of fitness can be achieved in as little as ten weeks with such easy forms of exercise as walking, bicycling, and gardening.

TREATMENTS USED

Conventional medicine: Responses and observations:

Herbal medicine: Responses and observations:

Homeopathic medicine: Responses and observations:

Diet/nutritional supplements: Responses and observations:

Other treatments/measures: Responses and observations:

Follow-up Questions and Observations

Name: .... Date: ....

Symptoms and questions (be as specific as possible): ....

....

....

HEALTH-CARE VISIT

Practitioner consulted: ....

Tests and screening procedures performed, if any: ....

     Test (specify) ....

     Result ....

     Test (specify) ....

     Result ....

     Test (specify) ....

     Result ....

Treatments administered during the visit, if any: ....

....

Practitioner's observations/recommendations/answers to questions: ....

....

TREATMENTS USED

Conventional medicine: ....   Responses and observations: ....

....

....

Herbal medicine: ....   Responses and observations: ....

....

....

Homeopathic medicine: ....   Responses and observations: ....

....

....

Diet/nutritional supplements: ....   Responses and observations: ....

....

....

Other treatments/measures: ....   Responses and observations: ....

....

....

Follow-up Questions and Observations ....

....

....

Name: .... Date: ....

Symptoms and questions (be as specific as possible): ....

....

....

HEALTH-CARE VISIT

Practitioner consulted: ....

Tests and screening procedures performed, if any: ....

    Test (specify) ....

    Result ....

    Test (specify) ....

    Result ....

    Test (specify) ....

    Result ....

Treatments administered during the visit, if any: ....

....

Practitioner's observations/recommendations/answers to questions: ....

....

....

TREATMENTS USED

Conventional medicine:	Responses and observations:
Herbal medicine:	Responses and observations:
Homeopathic medicine:	Responses and observations:
Diet/nutritional supplements:	Responses and observations:
Other treatments/measures:	Responses and observations:

Follow-up Questions and Observations ....

....

....

Name: .... Date: ....

Symptoms and questions (be as specific as possible):

....

....

....

Health Spotlight: Nasal Saline Flush

Nasal saline flushes cleanse the sinuses and the tissues that line the nasal passages, as well as soothing the mucous membranes and thinning mucus. They are very useful in the treatment of respiratory allergies and sinus infections. Dissolve ¼ teaspoon of salt and ⅛ teaspoon of baking soda in 4 ounces of water. Spray the mixture inside your nose with a bulb syringe or instill several drops into your nose with an eyedropper. If you are using this technique to clear nasal congestion, you can then suck out the mucus with a bulb syringe. If you are using it to soothe and moisten the mucous membranes, do not suction out mucus afterward.

HEALTH-CARE VISIT

Practitioner consulted: ....

Tests and screening procedures performed, if any:

Test (specify) ....

Result ....

Test (specify) ....

Result ....

Test (specify) ....

Result ....

Treatments administered during the visit, if any:

....

Practitioner's observations/recommendations/answers to questions:

....

TREATMENTS USED

Conventional medicine: .... Responses and observations: ....

....

Herbal medicine: .... Responses and observations: ....

....

Homeopathic medicine: .... Responses and observations: ....

....

Diet/nutritional supplements: .... Responses and observations: ....

....

Other treatments/measures: .... Responses and observations: ....

....

....

Follow-up Questions and Observations

....

....

....

Name: ....   Date: ....

Symptoms and questions (be as specific as possible): ....

....

....

HEALTH-CARE VISIT

Practitioner consulted: ....

Tests and screening procedures performed, if any:

    Test (specify) ....

    Result ....

    Test (specify) ....

    Result ....

    Test (specify) ....

    Result ....

Treatments administered during the visit, if any: ....

....

Practitioner's observations/recommendations/answers to questions: ....

....

....

TREATMENTS USED

Conventional medicine:	Responses and observations:
Herbal medicine:	Responses and observations:
Homeopathic medicine:	Responses and observations:
Diet/nutritional supplements:	Responses and observations:
Other treatments/measures:	Responses and observations:

Follow-up Questions and Observations ....

....

....

Health Spotlight: Barley Water

Barley water is a traditional home remedy that is particularly good at supporting recovery from illness or surgery if you are not yet up to eating solid foods. Add 1 cup of barley to 4 cups of water in a large glass, enameled, or stainless-steel saucepan, and bring to a boil over medium heat. Reduce the heat to a simmer and cook, covered or uncovered, for one hour. Remove the pot from the heat, strain out the grain, and drink the resulting broth in small sips throughout the day. You can drink it either warm or cool, as you prefer. If you dislike the taste of barley, you can substitute an equal amount of brown rice.

Name: .... Date: ....

Symptoms and questions (be as specific as possible): ....

....

....

HEALTH-CARE VISIT

Practitioner consulted: ....

Tests and screening procedures performed, if any:

    Test (specify) ....

    Result ....

    Test (specify) ....

    Result ....

    Test (specify) ....

    Result ....

Treatments administered during the visit, if any: ....

....

Practitioner's observations/recommendations/answers to questions: ....

....

....

TREATMENTS USED

Conventional medicine:	Responses and observations:
Herbal medicine:	Responses and observations:
Homeopathic medicine:	Responses and observations:
Diet/nutritional supplements:	Responses and observations:
Other treatments/measures:	Responses and observations:

Follow-up Questions and Observations ....

....

....

Name: .... Date: ....

Symptoms and questions (be as specific as possible): ....

....

....

....

HEALTH-CARE VISIT

Practitioner consulted: ....

Tests and screening procedures performed, if any: ....

    Test (specify) ....

    Result ....

    Test (specify) ....

    Result ....

    Test (specify) ....

    Result ....

Treatments administered during the visit, if any: ....

....

Practitioner's observations/recommendations/answers to questions: ....

....

....

TREATMENTS USED

Conventional medicine: .... Responses and observations: ....

....

....

Herbal medicine: .... Responses and observations: ....

....

....

Homeopathic medicine: .... Responses and observations: ....

....

....

Diet/nutritional supplements: .... Responses and observations: ....

....

....

Other treatments/measures: .... Responses and observations: ....

....

....

Follow-up Questions and Observations ....

....

....

Name: .... Date: ....

Symptoms and questions (be as specific as possible):

....

....

....

Health Spotlight: Antioxidants

Free radicals are atoms, molecules, or fragments of molecules that are highly unstable and are ready to react with other atoms or molecules in their vicinity. Because they join so readily with other substances, free radicals can attack cells and cause damage to the body at the cellular level. They thus can contribute to many degenerative diseases as well as to the aging process. Exposure to free radicals is inevitable; they come from many sources, including normal metabolism as well as exposure to radiation, pollutants, and high levels of dietary fat, especially fats that have been subjected to heat. Substances that defuse free radicals are known as antioxidants. Antioxidants include nutrients, enzymes, and other substances. Antioxidant nutrients include beta-carotene, vitamin C, vitamin E, all carotenoids such as selenium, and the amino acid glutathione. Antioxidant enzymes include superoxide dismutase (SOD), peroxidase, and catalase. Many herbs also have antioxidant properties, among them bilberry, black currant, hawthorn, and turmeric.

HEALTH-CARE VISIT

Practitioner consulted: ....

Tests and screening procedures performed, if any:

Test (specify) ....

Result ....

Test (specify) ....

Result ....

Test (specify) ....

Result ....

Treatments administered during the visit, if any:

....

Practitioner's observations/recommendations/answers to questions:

....

....

TREATMENTS USED

Conventional medicine:	Responses and observations:
Herbal medicine:	Responses and observations:
Homeopathic medicine:	Responses and observations:
Diet/nutritional supplements:	Responses and observations:
Other treatments/measures:	Responses and observations:

Follow-up Questions and Observations

....

....

....

Name: .... Date: ....

Symptoms and questions (be as specific as possible): ....

....

....

HEALTH-CARE VISIT

Practitioner consulted: ....

Tests and screening procedures performed, if any:

    Test (specify) ....

    Result ....

    Test (specify) ....

    Result ....

    Test (specify) ....

    Result ....

Treatments administered during the visit, if any: ....

....

Practitioner's observations/recommendations/answers to questions: ....

....

....

TREATMENTS USED

Conventional medicine: ....

....

Responses and observations: ....

....

Herbal medicine: ....

....

Responses and observations: ....

....

Homeopathic medicine: ....

....

Responses and observations: ....

....

Diet/nutritional supplements: ....

....

Responses and observations: ....

....

Other treatments/measures: ....

....

Responses and observations: ....

....

Follow-up Questions and Observations ....

....

....

Name: .... Date: ....

Symptoms and questions (be as specific as possible): ....

....

....

HEALTH-CARE VISIT

Practitioner consulted: ....

Tests and screening procedures performed, if any: ....

     Test (specify) ....

     Result ....

     Test (specify) ....

     Result ....

     Test (specify) ....

     Result ....

Treatments administered during the visit, if any: ....

....

Practitioner's observations/recommendations/answers to questions: ....

....

....

TREATMENTS USED

Conventional medicine:	Responses and observations:
....	....
Herbal medicine:	Responses and observations:
....	....
Homeopathic medicine:	Responses and observations:
....	....
Diet/nutritional supplements:	Responses and observations:
....	....
Other treatments/measures:	Responses and observations:
....	....

Follow-up Questions and Observations

....

....

....

Name: .... Date: ....

Symptoms and questions (be as specific as possible): ....

....

....

HEALTH-CARE VISIT

Practitioner consulted: ....

Tests and screening procedures performed, if any:

    Test (specify) ....

    Result ....

    Test (specify) ....

    Result ....

    Test (specify) ....

    Result ....

Treatments administered during the visit, if any: ....

....

Practitioner's observations/recommendations/answers to questions: ....

....

....

TREATMENTS USED

Conventional medicine: .... Responses and observations: ....

....

....

Herbal medicine: .... Responses and observations: ....

....

....

Homeopathic medicine: .... Responses and observations: ....

....

....

Diet/nutritional supplements: .... Responses and observations: ....

....

....

Other treatments/measures: .... Responses and observations: ....

....

....

Follow-up Questions and Observations

....

....

....

Name: .... Date: ....

Symptoms and questions (be as specific as possible): ....

....

....

Health Spotlight: Cancer

- Cancer is not a single disease, but rather a broad category of illnesses. What they have in common is the uncontrolled growth of certain cells in the body.

- A cancerous tumor can develop in any part of the body, but they are more likely to occur in certain types of tissues than in others.

- Among men, the most common type of cancer is prostate cancer; among women, the most common type is breast cancer. For people of both sexes, however, the deadliest form of cancer is lung cancer.

- An inherited predisposition or genetic condition can increase the possibility of developing cancer. For example, people with Down syndrome have a greater risk of developing leukemia than other people do.

HEALTH-CARE VISIT

Practitioner consulted: ....

Tests and screening procedures performed, if any:

    Test (specify) ....

    Result ....

    Test (specify) ....

    Result ....

    Test (specify) ....

    Result ....

Treatments administered during the visit, if any: ....

Practitioner's observations/recommendations/answers to questions: ....

....

TREATMENTS USED

Conventional medicine: .... Responses and observations: ....

....

Herbal medicine: .... Responses and observations: ....

....

Homeopathic medicine: .... Responses and observations: ....

....

Diet/nutritional supplements: .... Responses and observations: ....

....

Other treatments/measures: .... Responses and observations: ....

....

....

Follow-up Questions and Observations

....

....

Name: .... Date: ....

Symptoms and questions (be as specific as possible): ....

....

....

HEALTH-CARE VISIT

Practitioner consulted: ....

Tests and screening procedures performed, if any:

    Test (specify) ....

    Result ....

    Test (specify) ....

    Result ....

    Test (specify) ....

    Result ....

Treatments administered during the visit, if any: ....

....

Practitioner's observations/recommendations/answers to questions: ....

....

- Some types of cancer appear to have an infectious origin. For example, infection with sexually transmitted papillomavirus, which causes genital warts, can lead to cervical cancer; a hepatitis C infection can lead to liver cancer.

- Different medical terms are used to describe different types of cancers. The basic categories of cancer include carcinomas (including many cancers of the skin, mucous membranes, glands, and internal organs), leukemia (cancers of the blood-cell—forming tissues), lymphoma (cancers of lymphatic tissue), and sarcoma (primarily cancers of the bones, muscles, and connective tissues).

TREATMENTS USED

Conventional medicine: ....

....

Responses and observations: ....

....

Herbal medicine: ....

....

Responses and observations: ....

....

Homeopathic medicine: ....

....

Responses and observations: ....

....

Diet/nutritional supplements: ....

....

Responses and observations: ....

....

Other treatments/measures: ....

....

....

Responses and observations: ....

....

....

Follow-up Questions and Observations

....

....

Name: .... Date: ....

Symptoms and questions (be as specific as possible): ....

....

....

HEALTH-CARE VISIT

Practitioner consulted: ....

Tests and screening procedures performed, if any:

    Test (specify) ....

    Result ....

    Test (specify) ....

    Result ....

    Test (specify) ....

    Result ....

Treatments administered during the visit, if any: ....

....

Practitioner's observations/recommendations/answers to questions: ......

....

....

TREATMENTS USED

Conventional medicine: .... | Responses and observations: ....

.... | ....

Herbal medicine: .... | Responses and observations: ....

.... | ....

Homeopathic medicine: .... | Responses and observations: ....

.... | ....

Diet/nutritional supplements: .... | Responses and observations: ....

.... | ....

Other treatments/measures: .... | Responses and observations: ....

.... | ....

.... | ....

Follow-up Questions and Observations ....

....

....

Name: .... Date: ....

Symptoms and questions (be as specific as possible): ....

....

....

HEALTH-CARE VISIT

Practitioner consulted: ....

Tests and screening procedures performed, if any:

    Test (specify) ....

    Result ....

    Test (specify) ....

    Result ....

    Test (specify) ....

    Result ....

Treatments administered during the visit, if any: ....

....

Practitioner's observations/recommendations/answers to questions: ....

....

....

TREATMENTS USED

Conventional medicine:	Responses and observations:
Herbal medicine:	Responses and observations:
Homeopathic medicine:	Responses and observations:
Diet/nutritional supplements:	Responses and observations:
Other treatments/measures:	Responses and observations:

Follow-up Questions and Observations ....

....

....

Name: .... Date: ....

Symptoms and questions (be as specific as possible):

....

....

....

HEALTH-CARE VISIT

Practitioner consulted: ....

Tests and screening procedures performed, if any:

Test (specify) ....

Result ....

Test (specify) ....

Result ....

Test (specify) ....

Result ....

Treatments administered during the visit, if any:

....

Practitioner's observations/recommendations/answers to questions:

....

....

Health Spotlight: The Different Seasons of Hay Fever

- Hay fever that recurs in spring is most often due to an allergy to pollens from grass and trees.

- Hay fever that occurs in the late summer and early fall is usually caused by sensitivity to ragweed pollen and molds.

- Unfortunately, it is possible to be allergic to more than one type of pollen, resulting in hay fever that persists for many months of the year.

TREATMENTS USED

Conventional medicine: .... Responses and observations: ....

....

Herbal medicine: .... Responses and observations: ....

....

Homeopathic medicine: .... Responses and observations: ....

....

Diet/nutritional supplements: .... Responses and observations: ....

....

Other treatments/measures: .... Responses and observations: ....

....

Follow-up Questions and Observations ....

....

....

Name: .... Date: ....

Symptoms and questions (be as specific as possible): ....

....

....

HEALTH-CARE VISIT

Practitioner consulted: ....

Tests and screening procedures performed, if any:

    Test (specify) ....

    Result ....

    Test (specify) ....

    Result ....

    Test (specify) ....

    Result ....

Treatments administered during the visit, if any: ....

....

Practitioner's observations/recommendations/answers to questions: ....

....

....

TREATMENTS USED

Conventional medicine:	Responses and observations:
....	....
....	....
Herbal medicine:	Responses and observations:
....	....
....	....
Homeopathic medicine:	Responses and observations:
....	....
....	....
Diet/nutritional supplements:	Responses and observations:
....	....
....	....
Other treatments/measures:	Responses and observations:
....	....
....	....

Follow-up Questions and Observations ....

....

....

Name: .... Date: ....

Symptoms and questions (be as specific as possible): ....

....

....

HEALTH-CARE VISIT

Practitioner consulted: ....

Tests and screening procedures performed, if any:

    Test (specify) ....

    Result ....

    Test (specify) ....

    Result ....

    Test (specify) ....

    Result ....

Treatments administered during the visit, if any: ....

....

Practitioner's observations/recommendations/answers to questions: ....

....

....

TREATMENTS USED

Conventional medicine: .... Responses and observations: ....

....

Herbal medicine: .... Responses and observations: ....

....

Homeopathic medicine: .... Responses and observations: ....

....

Diet/nutritional supplements: .... Responses and observations: ....

....

Other treatments/measures: .... Responses and observations: ....

....

....

Follow-up Questions and Observations ....

....

....

Name: .... Date: ....

Symptoms and questions (be as specific as possible): ....

....

....

HEALTH-CARE VISIT

Practitioner consulted: ....

Tests and screening procedures performed, if any:

    Test (specify) ....

    Result ....

    Test (specify) ....

    Result ....

    Test (specify) ....

    Result ....

Treatments administered during the visit, if any: ....

....

Practitioner's observations/recommendations/answers to questions: ....

....

....

TREATMENTS USED

Conventional medicine: ....   Responses and observations: ....

....

Herbal medicine: ....   Responses and observations: ....

....

Homeopathic medicine: ....   Responses and observations: ....

....

Diet/nutritional supplements: ....   Responses and observations: ....

....

Other treatments/measures: ....   Responses and observations: ....

....

....

Follow-up Questions and Observations

....

....

....

Name: .... Date: ....

Symptoms and questions (be as specific as possible): ....

....

....

HEALTH-CARE VISIT

Practitioner consulted: ....

Tests and screening procedures performed, if any:

    Test (specify) ....

    Result ....

    Test (specify) ....

    Result ....

    Test (specify) ....

    Result ....

Treatments administered during the visit, if any: ....

Practitioner's observations/recommendations/answers to questions: ....

....

....

TREATMENTS USED

Conventional medicine:	Responses and observations:
Herbal medicine:	Responses and observations:
Homeopathic medicine:	Responses and observations:
Diet/nutritional supplements:	Responses and observations:
Other treatments/measures:	Responses and observations:

Follow-up Questions and Observations ....

....

....

Name: .... Date: ....

Symptoms and questions (be as specific as possible): ....
....
....

HEALTH-CARE VISIT

Practitioner consulted: ....

Tests and screening procedures performed, if any:

    Test (specify) ....

    Result ....

    Test (specify) ....

    Result ....

    Test (specify) ....

    Result ....

Treatments administered during the visit, if any: ....
....

Practitioner's observations/recommendations/answers to questions: ....
....
....

TREATMENTS USED

Conventional medicine:	Responses and observations:
....	....
....	....
Herbal medicine:	Responses and observations:
....	....
....	....
Homeopathic medicine:	Responses and observations:
....	....
....	....
Diet/nutritional supplements:	Responses and observations:
....	....
....	....
Other treatments/measures:	Responses and observations:
....	....
....	....

Follow-up Questions and Observations
....
....
....

Health Spotlight: Fever

- Fever is usually defined as a body temperature at least 1°F above 98.6°F (37.0°C). However, body temperature actually can vary by as much as 2°F over the course of a day. When taken by mouth, body temperature is usually between 96.8°F and 99.4°F.

- Fever is part of the body's defense mechanism against infectious invaders; viruses and bacteria do not survive well in a body with an elevated temperature.

- There is generally no need to take measures to lower a temperature that is 102°F or under. In fact, it may even be helpful to leave it alone, since fever aids in fighting illness. It is a good idea to increase your intake of fluids, though, because fever can be dehydrating.

- A temperature over 102°F can cause discomfort on its own, regardless of the seriousness of what is causing it. In that case, bringing it down can help you feel better.

- Children generally are more prone to fever, and to high fever, than adults are. In addition, susceptibility to fever can vary a great deal from individual to individual.

Name: .... Date: ....

Symptoms and questions (be as specific as possible): ....

....

....

HEALTH-CARE VISIT

Practitioner consulted: ....

Tests and screening procedures performed, if any:

    Test (specify) ....

    Result ....

    Test (specify) ....

    Result ....

    Test (specify) ....

    Result ....

Treatments administered during the visit, if any: ....

....

Practitioner's observations/recommendations/answers to questions: ....

....

....

TREATMENTS USED

Conventional medicine: .... Responses and observations: ....

....

Herbal medicine: .... Responses and observations: ....

....

Homeopathic medicine: .... Responses and observations: ....

....

Diet/nutritional supplements: .... Responses and observations: ....

....

Other treatments/measures: .... Responses and observations: ....

....

Follow-up Questions and Observations

....

....

....

Name: .... Date: ....

Symptoms and questions (be as specific as possible):

....

....

HEALTH-CARE VISIT

Practitioner consulted:

....

Tests and screening procedures performed, if any:

    Test (specify) ....

    Result ....

    Test (specify) ....

    Result ....

    Test (specify) ....

    Result ....

Treatments administered during the visit, if any:

....

Practitioner's observations/recommendations/answers to questions:

....

....

....

TREATMENTS USED

Conventional medicine:	Responses and observations:
Herbal medicine:	Responses and observations:
Homeopathic medicine:	Responses and observations:
Diet/nutritional supplements:	Responses and observations:
Other treatments/measures:	Responses and observations:

Follow-up Questions and Observations

....

....

....

Name: .... Date: ....

Symptoms and questions (be as specific as possible):
....
....
....

Health Spotlight: Understanding "Prescriptionese"

Ever wonder what those strange marks and abbreviations your doctor scrawls on the prescription pad mean? The following is a decoding key to some of the most common:

- bid = "twice a day"

- hs = "hour of sleep" (that is, "at bedtime")

- mcg = "micrograms"

- mg = "milligrams"

- po = "by mouth"

- prn = "as needed"

- q = "every" (as in "every four hours")

- qid = "four times a day"

- tid = "three times a day"

HEALTH-CARE VISIT

Practitioner consulted: ....

Tests and screening procedures performed, if any:

Test (specify) ....

Result ....

Test (specify) ....

Result ....

Test (specify) ....

Result ....

Treatments administered during the visit, if any:
....
....

Practitioner's observations/recommendations/answers to questions:
....
....

TREATMENTS USED

Conventional medicine: ....
....
....

Responses and observations: ....
....

Herbal medicine: ....
....
....

Responses and observations: ....
....

Homeopathic medicine: ....
....
....

Responses and observations: ....
....

Diet/nutritional supplements: ....
....
....

Responses and observations: ....
....

Other treatments/measures: ....
....
....

Responses and observations: ....
....

Follow-up Questions and Observations
....
....
....

IMPORTANT DOCUMENTS

Use the pages that follow to attach originals of important documents, such as birth certificates, health-care proxy, test results, prescription inserts, and so on.

ATTACH
IMPORTANT
DOCUMENTS
TO THIS
PAGE

ATTACH
IMPORTANT
DOCUMENTS
TO THIS
PAGE

ATTACH
IMPORTANT
DOCUMENTS
TO THIS
PAGE

ATTACH
IMPORTANT
DOCUMENTS
TO THIS
PAGE

ATTACH
IMPORTANT
DOCUMENTS
TO THIS
PAGE

ATTACH
IMPORTANT
DOCUMENTS
TO THIS
PAGE

ATTACH
IMPORTANT
DOCUMENTS
TO THIS
PAGE

ATTACH
IMPORTANT
DOCUMENTS
TO THIS
PAGE

ATTACH
IMPORTANT
DOCUMENTS
TO THIS
PAGE

ATTACH
IMPORTANT
DOCUMENTS
TO THIS
PAGE

IMPORTANT NAMES AND NUMBERS

Use the table that follows to record the names, contact information, and other relevant facts about the health-care professionals you have consulted.

Name:

Type of practitioner:

Address:

Telephone:

Referred by:

First consulted on (date):

Name:

Type of practitioner:

Address:

Telephone:

Referred by:

First consulted on (date):

Name:

Type of practitioner:

Address:

Telephone:

Referred by:

First consulted on (date):

Name:

Type of practitioner:

Address:

Telephone:

Referred by:

First consulted on (date):

Name:

Type of practitioner:

Address:

Telephone:

Referred by:

First consulted on (date):

Name:

Type of practitioner:

Address:

Telephone:

Referred by:

First consulted on (date):

Name:

Type of practitioner:

Address:

Telephone:

Referred by:

First consulted on (date):

Name:

Type of practitioner:

Address:

Telephone:

Referred by:

First consulted on (date):

Name:

Type of practitioner:

Address:

Telephone:

Referred by:

First consulted on (date):

Name:

Type of practitioner:

Address:

Telephone:

Referred by:

First consulted on (date):

Name:

Type of practitioner:

Address:

Telephone:

Referred by:

First consulted on (date):

Name:

Type of practitioner:

Address:

Telephone:

Referred by:

First consulted on (date):

Name:

Type of practitioner:

Address:

Telephone:

Referred by:

First consulted on (date):

Name:

Type of practitioner:

Address:

Telephone:

Referred by:

First consulted on (date):

Name:

Type of practitioner:

Address:

Telephone:

Referred by:

First consulted on (date):

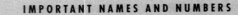

Name:

Type of practitioner:

Address:

Telephone:

Referred by:

First consulted on (date):

Name:

Type of practitioner:

Address:

Telephone:

Referred by:

First consulted on (date):

Name:

Type of practitioner:

Address:

Telephone:

Referred by:

First consulted on (date):

Name:

Type of practitioner:

Address:

Telephone:

Referred by:

First consulted on (date):

Name:

Type of practitioner:

Address:

Telephone:

Referred by:

First consulted on (date):

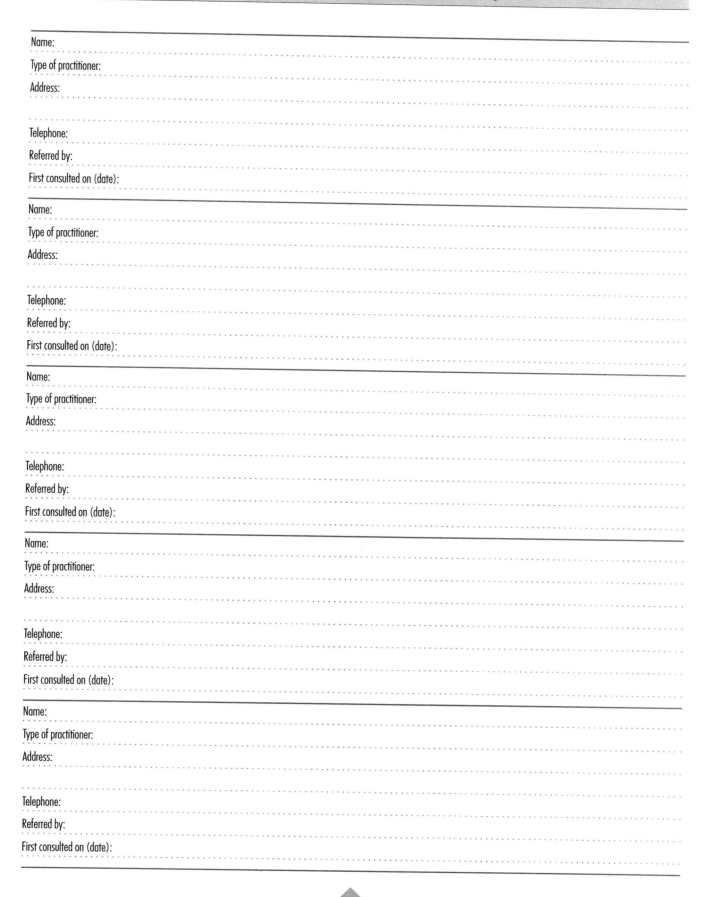

Name:

Type of practitioner:

Address:

Telephone:

Referred by:

First consulted on (date):

Name:

Type of practitioner:

Address:

Telephone:

Referred by:

First consulted on (date):

Name:

Type of practitioner:

Address:

Telephone:

Referred by:

First consulted on (date):

Name:

Type of practitioner:

Address:

Telephone:

Referred by:

First consulted on (date):

Name:

Type of practitioner:

Address:

Telephone:

Referred by:

First consulted on (date):

Name:

Type of practitioner:

Address:

Telephone:

Referred by:

First consulted on (date):

Name:

Type of practitioner:

Address:

Telephone:

Referred by:

First consulted on (date):

Name:

Type of practitioner:

Address:

Telephone:

Referred by:

First consulted on (date):

Name:

Type of practitioner:

Address:

Telephone:

Referred by:

First consulted on (date):

Name:

Type of practitioner:

Address:

Telephone:

Referred by:

First consulted on (date):